TCM Nutritional Therapy

Balancing Your Body and Mind

Mei Lin Zhang

Xspurts.com

A New Zealand Designed Product

Other Versions Available

Why limit yourself to just one format?

This book is now available in physical, digital, and audiobook options.

Choose the way you love to read and dive into the story today. You won't regret it!

Digital ISBN: 9781776968152
Physical ISBN: 9781776968145
Audio ISBN:

To obtain a different format of this book at a discounted price, please get in touch with us at:

http://isbn.xspurts.com/

Contents

Have Questions / Comments?

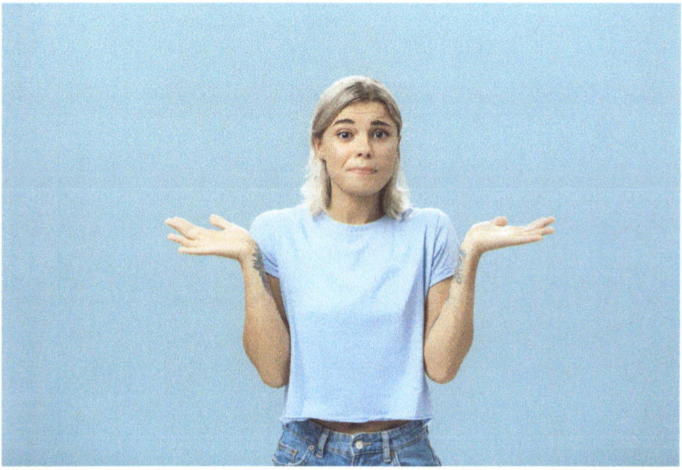

This book was designed to cover as much information as possible, but I know I have probably missed something, or some new amazing discovery has just come out.

If you notice something missing or have a question that I failed to answer, please get in touch and let me know. If I can, I will email you an answer and also update the book so others can also benefit from it.

Thanks For Being Awesome :)

Submit Your Questions / Comments At:

https://questions.xspurts.com

Get Free Stuff

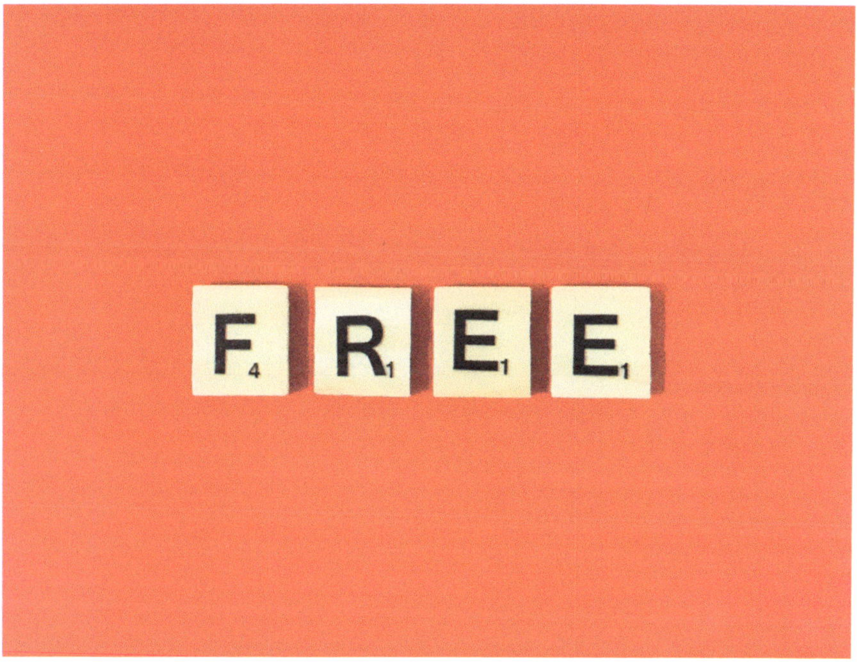

We love writing and have produced a huge number of books.

For being one of our amazing readers, we would love to offer you more books we have created, 100% free.

To claim this limited time special offer, simply go to the site below and enter your name and email address.

You will then receive loads (as we love our readers so much :) of our great books, content and audio direct to your email account, 100% free!

Get Loads of FREE Stuff at:

https://free.xspurts.com

Chapter One

Traditional Chinese Medicine (TCM) Nutrition: An Introduction

Traditional Chinese Medicine (TCM) is a system of medicine that has been practiced in China for thousands of years. It is based on the concept of Qi, which is the vital energy that flows through the body. According to TCM, Qi must flow smoothly and harmoniously for a person to be healthy. When Qi is blocked or unbalanced, it can lead to illness.

Nutrition is an important aspect of TCM. In TCM, food is not just a source of nutrients, but also a source of Qi. Different foods have different properties and can affect the body in different ways. By choosing the right foods, a person can balance their Qi and maintain good health.

TCM classifies foods into categories based on their properties. These categories include yin, yang, cold, hot, dry, damp, and neutral. Yin foods are cooling and moistening, while yang foods are warming and drying. Cold foods cool the body, while hot foods warm it up. Dry foods are dehydrating, while damp foods are moisturizing. Neutral foods have a balanced effect on the body.

According to TCM, a person's diet should be balanced and include foods from all categories. The proportion of each category of food should vary depending on a person's constitution, age, and health condition. For example, a person who tends to feel hot should eat more yin and cold foods, while a person who tends to feel cold should eat more yang and hot foods.

TCM also emphasizes the importance of eating seasonally and locally. In TCM, foods that are in season and grown locally are believed to be more nourishing and beneficial for the body. For example, in the summer, cooling foods such as watermelon and cucumber are recommended, while in the winter, warming foods such as ginger and cinnamon are recommended.

In addition to the properties of food, TCM also considers the energetic effects of cooking methods. Different cooking methods can affect the properties of food and its effect on the body. For example, stir-frying is a yang cooking method that can make yin foods more warming and drying. Boiling is a yin cooking method that can make yang foods more cooling and moistening.

TCM also considers the importance of eating mindfully and in a relaxed state. According to TCM, eating in a rushed or stressed state can affect digestion and the body's ability to absorb nutrients. TCM recommends eating in a calm and relaxed state and taking time to chew food thoroughly.

TCM also recommends specific foods and herbs for different health conditions. For example, ginger is commonly used in TCM to treat digestive issues and to warm the body. Goji berries are used to nourish the blood and improve vision. Turmeric is used to reduce inflammation and support liver health.

TCM also considers the concept of food energetics, which refers to the effect that foods have on the body beyond their nutritional content. For example, bitter foods such as dandelion greens are believed to stimulate digestion and cleanse the liver. Sweet foods such as honey are believed to nourish the spleen and calm the mind. Sour foods such as vinegar are believed to stimulate the appetite and promote digestion.

The principles of TCM nutrition

Traditional Chinese Medicine (TCM) is an ancient system of medicine that has been practiced in China for over two thousand years. TCM is based on the principle of balance, which is achieved through the harmonization of Qi, the vital energy that flows through the body. TCM nutrition is a key component of this system and is based on the principles of yin and yang, the five elements, and the Eight Principles.

Yin and Yang

In TCM, everything in the universe is classified as either yin or yang. Yin is associated with cold, dampness, and darkness, while yang is associated with warmth, dryness, and light. In the human body, yin and yang refer to the opposite yet complementary qualities that exist within us. The balance between yin and yang is essential for good health. TCM nutrition aims to maintain this balance through the selection of foods that are either yin or yang in nature.

For example, yang foods are warming and include foods such as ginger, garlic, and onions. These foods are beneficial for people who tend to feel cold or have a weak digestive system. Yin foods, on the other hand, are cooling and include foods such as watermelon, cucumber, and tofu. These foods are beneficial for people who tend to feel hot or have an excess of yang in their body.

The Five Elements

The Five Elements are wood, fire, earth, metal, and water. In TCM, each of these elements is associated with specific organs, emotions, and tastes. TCM nutrition aims to balance the Five Elements through the selection of foods that correspond to each element.

For example, wood is associated with the liver and gallbladder and is associated with the taste of sour. Foods that are beneficial for the liver and gallbladder include sour fruits such as lemons and limes, as well as green leafy vegetables such as kale and spinach.

Fire is associated with the heart and small intestine and is associated with the taste of bitter. Foods that are beneficial for the heart and small intestine include bitter vegetables such as dandelion greens and arugula, as well as bitter fruits such as grapefruit and cranberries.

Earth is associated with the spleen and stomach and is associated with the taste of sweet. Foods that are beneficial for the spleen and stomach include sweet vegetables such as sweet potatoes and carrots, as well as sweet fruits such as apples and pears.

Metal is associated with the lungs and large intestine and is associated with the taste of pungent. Foods that are beneficial for the lungs and large intestine include pungent vegetables such as onions and garlic, as well as pungent herbs such as ginger and turmeric.

Water is associated with the kidneys and bladder and is associated with the taste of salty. Foods that are beneficial for the kidneys and bladder include salty vegetables such as seaweed and celery, as well as salty meats such as fish and shellfish.

The Eight Principles

The Eight Principles are a diagnostic system used in TCM to assess a person's health. The Eight Principles include yin and yang, hot and cold, interior and exterior, and excess and deficiency. TCM nutrition aims to balance the Eight Principles through the selection of foods that correspond to each principle.

For example, a person with an excess of heat in their body may benefit from foods that are cooling and moistening, such as watermelon and cucumber. A person with a deficiency of Qi may benefit from foods that are warming and tonifying, such as ginger and ginseng.

Cooking Methods

In addition to the properties of food, TCM nutrition also considers the energetic effects of cooking methods. Different cooking methods can affect the properties of food and its effect on the body. TCM recommends cooking methods that are appropriate for a person's constitution

How TCM nutrition differs from Western nutrition

Traditional Chinese Medicine (TCM) nutrition and Western nutrition are two very different approaches to food and health. While Western nutrition focuses on the nutrient content of food, TCM nutrition emphasizes the energetic properties of food and their effects on the body. Below we will explore the key differences between TCM nutrition and Western nutrition.

Energetic Properties of Food

One of the main differences between TCM nutrition and Western nutrition is the emphasis on the energetic properties of food. In TCM, food is not just a source of nutrients but also a source of Qi, the vital energy that flows through the body. Different foods have different properties, such as yin or yang, and can affect the body in different ways.

For example, in TCM, foods that are yin in nature, such as watermelon and cucumber, are believed to have a cooling effect on the body. In contrast, foods that are yang in nature, such as ginger and garlic, are believed to have a warming effect on the body. Western nutrition, on the other hand, does not consider the energetic properties of food and instead focuses on the nutrient content, such as protein, carbohydrates, and vitamins.

Individualized Approach

Another key difference between TCM nutrition and Western nutrition is the individualized approach. In TCM, the diet is tailored to the individual based on their constitution, age, and health condition. For example, a person who tends to feel cold may be advised to eat more warming foods, while a person who tends to feel hot may be advised to eat more cooling foods.

In contrast, Western nutrition tends to take a more general approach, with recommendations based on population-wide guidelines. While these guidelines can be helpful for the general population, they may not be appropriate for everyone. TCM nutrition recognizes that each person is unique and requires an individualized approach to achieve optimal health.

Seasonal Eating

TCM nutrition also emphasizes the importance of seasonal eating. In TCM, foods that are in season and grown locally are believed to be more nourishing and beneficial for the body. For example, in the summer, cooling foods such as watermelon and cucumber are recommended, while in the winter, warming foods such as ginger and cinnamon are recommended.

Western nutrition, on the other hand, tends to focus on the availability of food year-round and often overlooks the importance of seasonal eating. This can result in a diet that is not in harmony with the changing seasons and may not provide the optimal nutrients for each season.

Food as Medicine

In TCM, food is considered a form of medicine. Specific foods and herbs are recommended for different health conditions, and the diet is tailored to the individual's health needs. For example, ginger is commonly used in TCM to treat digestive issues and to warm the body. Goji berries are used to nourish the blood and improve vision. Turmeric is used to reduce inflammation and support liver health.

In Western nutrition, while there is recognition of the role of nutrition in disease prevention and management, there is less emphasis on using food as medicine. Instead, medications and supplements are often used to treat specific health conditions.

Cooking Methods

TCM nutrition also considers the energetic effects of cooking methods. Different cooking methods can affect the properties of food and its effect on the body. TCM recommends cooking methods that are appropriate for a person's constitution. For example, stir-frying is a yang cooking method that can make yin foods more warming and drying. Boiling is a yin cooking method that can make yang foods more cooling and moistening.

In Western nutrition, cooking methods are often based on taste preference and convenience rather than their energetic effects on the body.

Chapter Two

The Five Elements and Their Corresponding Tastes

Traditional Chinese Medicine (TCM) has a unique approach to nutrition that is based on the principles of Yin and Yang, the Five Elements, and the Eight Principles. In TCM, the Five Elements - wood, fire, earth, metal, and water - are believed to represent the fundamental building blocks of the universe, and each element corresponds to specific organs, emotions, and tastes. Below we will explore the Five Elements and their corresponding tastes in TCM nutrition.

Wood Element - Sour Taste

The wood element is associated with the liver and gallbladder and is associated with the sour taste. Sour foods are believed to promote the flow of Qi, the vital energy that flows through the body. Sour foods are also believed to help the liver and gallbladder function properly.

Examples of sour foods include lemons, limes, grapefruit, sour apples, and pickles. Sour flavors can also be found in foods such as sauerkraut, vinegar, and fermented foods.

Fire Element - Bitter Taste

The fire element is associated with the heart and small intestine and is associated with the bitter taste. Bitter foods are believed to stimulate digestion and help the body detoxify. Bitter foods are also believed to calm the mind and promote heart health.

Examples of bitter foods include dark leafy greens such as kale, collard greens, and dandelion greens. Other examples include bitter melon, grapefruit, and bitter herbs such as chamomile, dandelion, and goldenseal.

Earth Element - Sweet Taste

The earth element is associated with the spleen and stomach and is associated with the sweet taste. Sweet foods are believed to nourish the body and provide energy. Sweet foods are also believed to support the digestive system and help the body absorb nutrients.

Examples of sweet foods include sweet potatoes, carrots, winter squash, yams, and beets. Fruits such as apples, pears, dates, and raisins are also considered sweet.

Metal Element - Pungent Taste

The metal element is associated with the lungs and large intestine and is associated with the pungent taste. Pungent foods are believed to promote circulation and help the body eliminate toxins. Pungent foods are also believed to stimulate the appetite and promote digestion.

Examples of pungent foods include onions, garlic, ginger, horseradish, and peppers. Pungent herbs such as cumin, fennel, and coriander are also considered pungent.

Water Element - Salty Taste

The water element is associated with the kidneys and bladder and is associated with the salty taste. Salty foods are believed to promote hydration and help the body retain water. Salty foods are also believed to support the kidneys and help regulate blood pressure.

Examples of salty foods include seaweed, miso, soy sauce, and pickled vegetables. Processed and packaged foods, such as chips and crackers, are also considered salty.

In TCM nutrition, it is important to consume foods from all Five Elements in order to maintain balance and promote good health. By incorporating a variety of flavors into our diet, we can support our organs and promote the smooth flow of Qi. It is important to note that while TCM nutrition emphasizes the energetic properties of food, it is still important to consume a balanced and nutritious diet that meets our individual needs.

Wood: Sour

The Wood element is one of the Five Elements in Traditional Chinese Medicine (TCM) that corresponds to the liver and gallbladder. In TCM, the Wood element is also associated with the sour taste, which is believed to promote the flow of Qi, the vital energy that flows through the body. Below we will explore the role of the Wood element and the sour taste in TCM nutrition.

The Wood Element

In TCM, the Wood element is associated with growth, flexibility, and change. The liver and gallbladder are considered the organs of the Wood element, and they play a vital role in regulating the flow of Qi and blood in the body. The liver is responsible for detoxifying the blood, storing and releasing blood sugar, and regulating the flow of Qi, while the gallbladder stores and secretes bile, which aids in digestion.

When the Wood element is in balance, a person feels a sense of vitality and growth. However, when the Wood element is out of balance, a person may experience feelings of frustration, anger, or depression. TCM nutrition can play an important role in maintaining the balance of the Wood element.

The Sour Taste

In TCM, the sour taste is associated with the Wood element and is believed to have a contracting and consolidating effect on the body. The sour taste is believed to promote the flow of Qi and blood and to help the liver and gallbladder function properly.

Sour foods are also believed to help balance the body's pH level and to support the immune system. The sour taste is also believed to have an astringent effect, which can help to tighten and tone tissues in the body.

Examples of Sour Foods

In TCM nutrition, sour foods are believed to have a cooling effect on the body and are recommended for people with an excess of heat or a deficiency of Yin. Examples of sour foods include:

Citrus fruits such as lemons, limes, and oranges

Berries such as raspberries, strawberries, and cranberries

Fermented foods such as sauerkraut, kimchi, and pickles

Vinegar and other sour condiments

Tamarind, a sour fruit commonly used in Southeast Asian cooking

Incorporating Sour Foods into the Diet

Incorporating sour foods into the diet can be an effective way to support the Wood element and promote good health. One way to incorporate sour foods into the diet is to add fresh lemon or lime juice to water or tea.

Another way is to add a small amount of vinegar or lemon juice to salad dressings or marinades.

Fermented foods such as sauerkraut and kimchi can also be a good source of sour flavor. These foods are made by fermenting vegetables with salt and can be eaten as a side dish or added to sandwiches or wraps.

It is important to note that while sour foods are beneficial in moderation, consuming too many sour foods can be harmful to the body. In excess, sour foods can cause digestive upset, promote the growth of harmful bacteria, and damage tooth enamel. It is important to consume sour foods as part of a balanced diet and to consult with a qualified TCM practitioner before making any significant changes to the diet.

Fire: Bitter

In Traditional Chinese Medicine (TCM), the Fire element is associated with the heart and small intestine, and the bitter taste is associated with this element. In TCM, the Fire element represents passion, joy, and creativity, and the bitter taste is believed to promote digestion and detoxification. Below we will explore the role of the Fire element and the bitter taste in TCM nutrition.

The Fire Element

The Fire element is associated with the heart and small intestine in TCM. The heart is considered the ruler of the body and is responsible for circulating blood and regulating emotions. The small intestine is responsible for absorbing nutrients and separating the pure from the impure.

When the Fire element is in balance, a person feels a sense of joy and creativity. However, when the Fire element is out of balance, a person may experience feelings of anxiety, restlessness, or depression. TCM nutrition can play an important role in maintaining the balance of the Fire element.

The Bitter Taste

In TCM, the bitter taste is associated with the Fire element and is believed to promote digestion and detoxification. Bitter foods are believed to stimulate the production of digestive enzymes and bile, which aids in the digestion of fats. Bitter foods are also believed to have a purifying effect on the body, helping to remove toxins and promote healthy skin.

In addition, the bitter taste is believed to have a cooling effect on the body, which can help to reduce inflammation and calm the mind. The bitter taste is also believed to promote heart health, improving circulation and reducing the risk of heart disease.

Examples of Bitter Foods

In TCM nutrition, bitter foods are believed to have a drying effect on the body and are recommended for people with an excess of dampness or a deficiency of Yang. Examples of bitter foods include:

Dark leafy greens such as kale, collard greens, and spinach

Bitter melon, a fruit commonly used in Asian cooking

Citrus peels such as orange, lemon, and grapefruit zest

Cacao, the raw ingredient used to make chocolate

Bitter herbs such as dandelion, gentian, and milk thistle

Incorporating Bitter Foods into the Diet

Incorporating bitter foods into the diet can be an effective way to support the Fire element and promote good health. One way to incorporate bitter foods into the diet is to add dark leafy greens to salads or smoothies. Another way is to drink bitter herbal teas such as dandelion or chamomile tea.

Bitter foods can also be used as a seasoning in cooking. Adding citrus zest to marinades or using bitter herbs such as thyme or rosemary in recipes can add a delicious bitter flavor to dishes.

It is important to note that while bitter foods are beneficial in moderation, consuming too many bitter foods can be harmful to the body. In excess, bitter foods can cause digestive upset and may interfere with the absorption of nutrients. It is important to consume bitter foods as part of a balanced diet and to consult with a qualified TCM practitioner before making any significant changes to the diet.

Earth: Sweet

In Traditional Chinese Medicine (TCM), the Earth element is associated with the spleen and stomach, and the sweet taste is associated with this element. In TCM, the Earth element represents stability, grounding, and nourishment, and the sweet taste is believed to provide energy and support digestion. Below we will explore the role of the Earth element and the sweet taste in TCM nutrition.

The Earth Element

The Earth element is associated with the spleen and stomach in TCM. The spleen is responsible for transforming food into energy and regulating the blood. The stomach is responsible for breaking down food and extracting nutrients.

When the Earth element is in balance, a person feels a sense of stability and nourishment. However, when the Earth element is out of balance, a person may experience feelings of worry, anxiety, or fatigue. TCM nutrition can play an important role in maintaining the balance of the Earth element.

The Sweet Taste

In TCM, the sweet taste is associated with the Earth element and is believed to provide energy and support digestion. Sweet foods are believed to nourish the body and provide the energy needed for daily activities. Sweet foods are also believed to support the digestive system and help the body absorb nutrients.

In addition, the sweet taste is believed to have a moistening effect on the body, which can help to lubricate the tissues and promote healthy skin. The sweet taste is also believed to have a calming effect on the mind, reducing anxiety and promoting relaxation.

Examples of Sweet Foods

In TCM nutrition, sweet foods are believed to have a warming effect on the body and are recommended for people with an excess of cold or a deficiency of Qi. Examples of sweet foods include:

Sweet potatoes, carrots, and winter squash

Fruits such as apples, pears, dates, and raisins

Whole grains such as rice, oats, and barley

Legumes such as lentils, chickpeas, and kidney beans

Sweet herbs such as licorice root and cinnamon

Incorporating Sweet Foods into the Diet

Incorporating sweet foods into the diet can be an effective way to support the Earth element and promote good health. One way to incorporate sweet foods into the diet is to eat a variety of fruits and vegetables, which provide natural sweetness and are also rich in vitamins and minerals.

Another way is to choose complex carbohydrates such as whole grains, which provide sustained energy and also contain fiber to support digestion. Adding sweet herbs such as cinnamon or licorice root to teas or recipes can also provide a delicious sweet flavor.

It is important to note that while sweet foods are beneficial in moderation, consuming too many sweet foods can be harmful to the body. In excess, sweet foods can cause blood sugar imbalances and contribute to weight gain. It is important to consume sweet foods as part of a balanced diet and to consult with a qualified TCM practitioner before making any significant changes to the diet.

Metal: Pungent

In Traditional Chinese Medicine (TCM), the Metal element is associated with the lungs and large intestine, and the pungent taste is associated with this element. In TCM, the Metal element represents clarity, precision, and refinement, and the pungent taste is believed to promote the flow of Qi and aid in the elimination of toxins. Below we will explore the role of the Metal element and the pungent taste in TCM nutrition.

The Metal Element

The Metal element is associated with the lungs and large intestine in TCM. The lungs are responsible for breathing and regulating the flow of Qi, while the large intestine is responsible for eliminating waste and toxins from the body.

When the Metal element is in balance, a person feels a sense of clarity and precision. However, when the Metal element is out of balance, a person may experience feelings of grief, sadness, or detachment. TCM nutrition can play an important role in maintaining the balance of the Metal element.

The Pungent Taste

In TCM, the pungent taste is associated with the Metal element and is believed to promote the flow of Qi and aid in the elimination of toxins. Pungent foods are believed to stimulate the senses and promote circulation in the body. Pungent foods are also believed to have a warming effect on the body, which can help to reduce congestion and promote healthy respiration.

In addition, the pungent taste is believed to have a drying effect on the body, which can help to reduce excess mucus and phlegm. The pungent taste is also believed to promote mental clarity and alertness, improving focus and concentration.

Examples of Pungent Foods

In TCM nutrition, pungent foods are believed to have a warming effect on the body and are recommended for people with an excess of cold or a deficiency of Qi. Examples of pungent foods include:

Garlic, onions, and ginger

Hot peppers such as cayenne, jalapeno, and habanero

Spices such as cumin, coriander, and turmeric

Radishes, mustard greens, and horseradish

Seeds such as fennel, caraway, and anise

Incorporating Pungent Foods into the Diet

Incorporating pungent foods into the diet can be an effective way to support the Metal element and promote good health. One way to incorporate pungent foods into the diet is to add garlic, onions, or ginger to recipes for flavor and health benefits. Another way is to add hot peppers or spices to dishes for a delicious and warming flavor.

Pungent foods can also be used in herbal remedies or teas to promote respiratory health and mental clarity. For example, ginger tea can be made by steeping fresh ginger in hot water for several minutes.

It is important to note that while pungent foods are beneficial in moderation, consuming too many pungent foods can be harmful to the body. In excess, pungent foods can cause digestive upset and may aggravate certain conditions such as acid reflux or ulcers. It is important to consume pungent foods as part of a balanced diet and to consult with a qualified TCM practitioner before making any significant changes to the diet.

Water: Salty

In Traditional Chinese Medicine (TCM), the Water element is associated with the kidneys and bladder, and the salty taste is associated with this element. In TCM, the Water element represents fluidity, adaptability, and resilience, and the salty taste is believed to promote the balance of fluids and electrolytes in the body. Below we will explore the role of the Water element and the salty taste in TCM nutrition.

The Water Element

The Water element is associated with the kidneys and bladder in TCM. The kidneys are responsible for filtering waste and regulating the balance of fluids and electrolytes in the body. The bladder is responsible for storing and eliminating urine.

When the Water element is in balance, a person feels a sense of fluidity and adaptability. However, when the Water element is out of balance, a person may experience feelings of fear, insecurity, or lack of trust. TCM nutrition can play an important role in maintaining the balance of the Water element.

The Salty Taste

In TCM, the salty taste is associated with the Water element and is believed to promote the balance of fluids and electrolytes in the body. Salty foods are believed to promote hydration and help the body maintain the proper balance of sodium and potassium.

In addition, the salty taste is believed to have a grounding effect on the body, which can help to reduce anxiety and promote relaxation. The salty taste is also believed to support the health of the kidneys and promote healthy digestion.

Examples of Salty Foods

In TCM nutrition, salty foods are believed to have a cooling effect on the body and are recommended for people with an excess of heat or a deficiency of Yin. Examples of salty foods include:

Sea vegetables such as seaweed, kelp, and nori

Fish and shellfish such as salmon, shrimp, and oysters

Salted nuts or seeds such as almonds or sunflower seeds

Fermented foods such as miso, soy sauce, or pickles

Salt, in moderation

Incorporating Salty Foods into the Diet

Incorporating salty foods into the diet can be an effective way to support the Water element and promote good health. One way to incorporate salty foods into the diet is to add sea vegetables to soups or salads for a delicious and nutritious flavor.

Another way is to include fish or shellfish in meals for a source of healthy fats and protein. Salted nuts or seeds can also be used as a snack or added to recipes for flavor and health benefits.

It is important to note that while salty foods are beneficial in moderation, consuming too many salty foods can be harmful to the body. In excess, salty foods can contribute to high blood pressure and may aggravate certain conditions such as kidney disease or heart disease. It is important to consume salty foods as part of a balanced diet and to consult with a qualified TCM practitioner before making any significant changes to the diet.

Chapter Three

Yin and Yang in TCM Nutrition

In Traditional Chinese Medicine (TCM), the concept of Yin and Yang is used to describe the balance and harmony of opposing forces in the body. This principle applies to TCM nutrition as well, as different foods and flavors can be classified as either Yin or Yang. Below we will explore the role of Yin and Yang in TCM nutrition.

The Concept of Yin and Yang

The concept of Yin and Yang is rooted in the Taoist philosophy of ancient China. Yin and Yang are opposite yet complementary forces that exist in everything in the universe, including the human body. Yin represents qualities such as coldness, darkness, and moisture, while Yang represents qualities such as heat, light, and dryness. In TCM, the balance and harmony of Yin and Yang in the body is essential for good health.

In TCM nutrition, foods and flavors can be classified as either Yin or Yang. Foods that are classified as Yin are believed to be cooling and nourishing to the body, while foods that are classified as Yang are believed to be warming and stimulating to the body. The balance of Yin and Yang in the diet is important for maintaining the overall balance and harmony of Yin and Yang in the body.

Examples of Yin Foods

Yin foods are believed to be cooling and nourishing to the body, and are recommended for people with an excess of heat or a deficiency of Yin. Examples of Yin foods include:

Fruits such as watermelon, cucumber, and berries

Vegetables such as lettuce, celery, and sprouts

Sea vegetables such as seaweed and kelp

Herbal teas such as mint or chamomile

Dairy products such as milk and yogurt

Examples of Yang Foods

Yang foods are believed to be warming and stimulating to the body, and are recommended for people with an excess of cold or a deficiency of Yang. Examples of Yang foods include:

Meats such as beef, lamb, and chicken

Spices such as ginger, garlic, and cinnamon

Root vegetables such as carrots, onions, and potatoes

Grains such as quinoa, millet, and barley

Nuts and seeds such as almonds, pumpkin seeds, and walnuts

Balancing Yin and Yang in the Diet

In TCM nutrition, balancing Yin and Yang in the diet is important for maintaining good health. One way to balance Yin and Yang in the diet is to consume a variety of foods from both categories. For example, a meal might include a Yin salad with lettuce, cucumber, and sprouts, paired with a Yang dish of grilled chicken and root vegetables.

Another way to balance Yin and Yang in the diet is to consume foods that are neutral in nature, such as brown rice, whole grains, and some vegetables. Neutral foods do not have a strong Yin or Yang nature, and can help to balance the overall Yin and Yang balance in the body.

It is important to note that while the concept of Yin and Yang can be helpful in understanding the balance of opposing forces in the body, it is not a rigid system. Foods can have varying degrees of Yin and Yang nature, and the needs of each individual may be different based on their constitution and health concerns. It is important to consult with a qualified TCM practitioner to determine the best diet for each individual.

The concept of Yin and Yang

The concept of Yin and Yang is a central principle in Traditional Chinese Medicine (TCM), describing the balance of opposing forces in the universe and in the human body. This concept is applicable to TCM nutrition, where foods and flavors are classified as either Yin or Yang based on their properties and effects on the body. Below we will explore the concept of Yin and Yang and its relevance to TCM nutrition.

The Concept of Yin and Yang

The concept of Yin and Yang is rooted in the Taoist philosophy of ancient China. Yin and Yang are opposing yet complementary forces that exist in everything in the universe, including the human body. Yin represents qualities such as coldness, darkness, and moisture, while Yang represents qualities such as heat, light, and dryness. According to TCM, the balance and harmony of Yin and Yang in the body is essential for good health.

In TCM, the concept of Yin and Yang is used to describe various aspects of the body, such as the organs, meridians, and emotions. The balance of

Yin and Yang in these aspects is essential for maintaining good health and preventing disease.

Yin and Yang in TCM Nutrition

In TCM nutrition, foods and flavors are classified as either Yin or Yang based on their properties and effects on the body. Foods that are classified as Yin are believed to be cooling and nourishing to the body, while foods that are classified as Yang are believed to be warming and stimulating to the body. The balance of Yin and Yang in the diet is important for maintaining the overall balance and harmony of Yin and Yang in the body.

Yin Foods

Yin foods are believed to be cooling and nourishing to the body, and are recommended for people with an excess of heat or a deficiency of Yin. Examples of Yin foods include:

Fruits such as watermelon, cucumber, and berries

Vegetables such as lettuce, celery, and sprouts

Sea vegetables such as seaweed and kelp

Herbal teas such as mint or chamomile

Dairy products such as milk and yogurt

Yang Foods

Yang foods are believed to be warming and stimulating to the body, and are recommended for people with an excess of cold or a deficiency of Yang. Examples of Yang foods include:

Meats such as beef, lamb, and chicken

Spices such as ginger, garlic, and cinnamon

Root vegetables such as carrots, onions, and potatoes

Grains such as quinoa, millet, and barley

Nuts and seeds such as almonds, pumpkin seeds, and walnuts

Balancing Yin and Yang in the Diet

In TCM nutrition, balancing Yin and Yang in the diet is important for maintaining good health. One way to balance Yin and Yang in the diet is to consume a variety of foods from both categories. Another way is to consume foods that are neutral in nature, such as brown rice, whole grains, and some vegetables. Neutral foods do not have a strong Yin or Yang nature, and can help to balance the overall Yin and Yang balance in the body.

It is important to note that the concept of Yin and Yang is not a rigid system. Foods can have varying degrees of Yin and Yang nature, and the needs of each individual may be different based on their constitution and health concerns. It is important to consult with a qualified TCM practitioner to determine the best diet for each individual.

Balancing Yin and Yang through diet

In Traditional Chinese Medicine (TCM), the concept of Yin and Yang describes the balance of opposing forces in the universe and in the human body. When it comes to TCM nutrition, balancing Yin and Yang through diet is an essential component of maintaining good health. Below we will explore the principles of TCM nutrition that can help to balance Yin and Yang in the diet.

The Principles of Yin and Yang in TCM Nutrition

Yin and Yang are opposing yet complementary forces that exist in everything in the universe, including the human body. In TCM nutrition, foods and flavors are classified as either Yin or Yang based on their properties and effects on the body.

Yin foods are believed to be cooling and nourishing to the body, while Yang foods are believed to be warming and stimulating to the body. The balance of Yin and Yang in the diet is important for maintaining the overall balance and harmony of Yin and Yang in the body.

The following principles can help to balance Yin and Yang through diet:

Eating a Variety of Foods

Eating a variety of foods can help to balance Yin and Yang in the diet. For example, a meal might include a Yin salad with lettuce, cucumber, and sprouts, paired with a Yang dish of grilled chicken and root vegetables.

By incorporating a range of Yin and Yang foods into the diet, you can help to maintain the overall balance of these opposing forces in the body.

Eating with the Seasons

Eating with the seasons can also help to balance Yin and Yang in the diet. In TCM, each season is associated with different elements and energies, and certain foods are more beneficial during specific seasons.

For example, in the summer, Yin foods such as watermelon and cucumber are recommended to cool the body and balance excess Yang energy. In the winter, Yang foods such as root vegetables and warming spices are recommended to nourish the body and balance excess Yin energy.

Balancing Acid and Alkaline Foods

Balancing acid and alkaline foods can also help to balance Yin and Yang in the diet. In TCM, the body is believed to function best in a slightly alkaline environment. However, many modern diets are high in acid-forming foods such as meat, dairy, and processed foods.

To balance the pH levels in the body and promote overall health, it is important to include alkaline-forming foods such as leafy greens, vegetables, and fruits in the diet.

Eating Mindfully

Eating mindfully can also help to balance Yin and Yang in the diet. In TCM, the way that food is prepared and consumed can have an impact on its Yin and Yang nature.

For example, eating slowly and mindfully can help to promote the Yin nature of food by allowing the body to fully absorb and digest the nutrients. On the other hand, consuming food quickly and mindlessly can promote the Yang nature of food by stimulating the body and causing it to work harder to digest the food.

Consulting with a TCM Practitioner

Finally, consulting with a qualified TCM practitioner can help to determine the best diet for your individual needs. TCM practitioners can use diagnostic tools such as tongue and pulse diagnosis to assess your individual constitution and health concerns, and make dietary recommendations based on your specific needs.

Chapter Four

The Energetic Properties of Foods

In Traditional Chinese Medicine (TCM), the energetic properties of foods are a crucial aspect of TCM nutrition. Different foods have different energetic properties, which can affect the balance of Yin and Yang in the body. Below we will explore the energetic properties of foods in TCM nutrition.

The Five Flavors

1. In TCM, foods are classified into five flavors: sweet, sour, bitter, pungent, and salty. Each flavor is associated with different energetic properties, which can affect the balance of Yin and Yang in the body.

Sweet foods are believed to have a Yin nature, and are nourishing and moistening to the body. Examples of sweet foods include grains, fruits, and root vegetables.

Sour foods are believed to have a Yin nature, and are astringent and cooling to the body. Examples of sour foods include citrus fruits, vinegar, and fermented foods.

Bitter foods are believed to have a Yang nature, and are drying and cooling to the body. Examples of bitter foods include dark leafy greens, coffee, and dark chocolate.

Pungent foods are believed to have a Yang nature, and are warming and stimulating to the body. Examples of pungent foods include ginger, garlic, and chili peppers.

Salty foods are believed to have a Yang nature, and are astringent and warming to the body. Examples of salty foods include seaweed, miso, and soy sauce.

Balancing the Five Flavors

In TCM nutrition, balancing the five flavors is essential for maintaining the overall balance of Yin and Yang in the body. Consuming a variety of flavors can help to achieve this balance.

For example, if a meal is predominantly sweet, adding a sour or bitter flavor can help to balance the Yin nature of the meal. Likewise, if a meal is predominantly bitter or pungent, adding a sweet or salty flavor can help to balance the Yang nature of the meal.

Individual Differences

It is important to note that the energetic properties of foods can affect individuals differently based on their constitution and health concerns. For example, someone with excess heat may benefit from consuming more cooling, Yin foods, while someone with excess cold may benefit from consuming more warming, Yang foods.

It is important to consult with a qualified TCM practitioner to determine the best diet for your individual needs.

Cooking Methods

In addition to the flavor of foods, the cooking method can also affect the energetic properties of foods. For example, steaming or boiling can help to retain the Yin nature of foods, while roasting or grilling can increase the Yang nature of foods.

Cooking methods that use slow, low heat can help to retain the Yin nature of foods, while cooking methods that use high heat can increase the Yang nature of foods.

Hot, warm, neutral, cool, and cold foods

In Traditional Chinese Medicine (TCM), the temperature of foods is an important aspect of TCM nutrition. Different foods have different temperature properties, which can affect the balance of Yin and Yang in the body. Below we will explore the temperature properties of foods in TCM nutrition.

Hot and Warm Foods

Hot and warm foods are believed to have a Yang nature, and can be stimulating and energizing to the body. Examples of hot and warm foods include spices such as cinnamon, cloves, and ginger, as well as hot drinks such as coffee and tea.

Consuming too many hot and warm foods can lead to excess Yang energy in the body, which can manifest as symptoms such as dryness, inflammation, and agitation.

Neutral Foods

Neutral foods are believed to have a balanced Yin and Yang nature, and are neither cooling nor warming to the body. Examples of neutral foods include grains, legumes, and some fruits and vegetables.

In TCM, neutral foods are considered to be beneficial for maintaining the overall balance of Yin and Yang in the body.

Cool and Cold Foods

Cool and cold foods are believed to have a Yin nature, and can be cooling and calming to the body. Examples of cool and cold foods include fruits such as watermelon and citrus, as well as leafy greens and cucumbers.

Consuming too many cool and cold foods can lead to excess Yin energy in the body, which can manifest as symptoms such as lethargy, coldness, and dampness.

Balancing Temperature Properties of Foods

In TCM nutrition, balancing the temperature properties of foods is essential for maintaining the overall balance of Yin and Yang in the body. Consuming a variety of foods with different temperature properties can help to achieve this balance.

For example, if a meal is predominantly hot and warm, adding some neutral or cool foods can help to balance the Yang nature of the meal. Likewise, if a meal is predominantly cool or cold, adding some neutral or warm foods can help to balance the Yin nature of the meal.

Individual Differences

It is important to note that the temperature properties of foods can affect individuals differently based on their constitution and health concerns. For example, someone with excess heat may benefit from consuming more cooling, Yin foods, while someone with excess cold may benefit from consuming more warming, Yang foods.

It is important to consult with a qualified TCM practitioner to determine the best diet for your individual needs.

Cooking Methods

In addition to the temperature of foods, the cooking method can also affect the temperature properties of foods. For example, cooking methods that use high heat can increase the Yang nature of foods, while cooking methods that use low heat can increase the Yin nature of foods.

Steaming, boiling, and stewing are cooking methods that can help to retain the Yin nature of foods, while roasting, grilling, and frying can increase the Yang nature of foods.

The impact of food properties on the body

In Traditional Chinese Medicine (TCM), the properties of foods are believed to have a significant impact on the body. Different foods have different properties, including flavor, temperature, and energetic nature, which can affect the balance of Yin and Yang in the body. Below we will explore the impact of food properties on the body in TCM nutrition.

Flavor

The flavor of foods is an important aspect of TCM nutrition. Each flavor is associated with different energetic properties, which can affect the balance of Yin and Yang in the body.

For example, sweet foods are believed to have a Yin nature, and are nourishing and moistening to the body. On the other hand, bitter foods are believed to have a Yang nature, and are drying and cooling to the body.

By incorporating a variety of flavors into the diet, it is possible to achieve a balance of Yin and Yang in the body.

Temperature

The temperature of foods is another important aspect of TCM nutrition. Different foods have different temperature properties, which can affect the balance of Yin and Yang in the body.

For example, hot and warm foods are believed to have a Yang nature, and can be stimulating and energizing to the body. On the other hand, cool and cold foods are believed to have a Yin nature, and can be cooling and calming to the body.

By balancing the temperature properties of foods in the diet, it is possible to maintain the overall balance of Yin and Yang in the body.

Energetic Nature

The energetic nature of foods is also an important aspect of TCM nutrition. Each food is believed to have a specific energetic nature, which can affect the balance of Yin and Yang in the body.

For example, Yin foods are believed to be cooling and nourishing to the body, while Yang foods are believed to be warming and stimulating to the body.

By balancing the Yin and Yang nature of foods in the diet, it is possible to maintain the overall balance of Yin and Yang in the body.

Individual Differences

It is important to note that the impact of food properties on the body can vary from person to person based on individual constitution and health concerns.

For example, someone with excess heat may benefit from consuming more cooling, Yin foods, while someone with excess cold may benefit from consuming more warming, Yang foods.

It is important to consult with a qualified TCM practitioner to determine the best diet for your individual needs.

Overall Impact

The impact of food properties on the body in TCM nutrition is significant. By balancing the flavor, temperature, and energetic nature of foods in the diet, it is possible to maintain the overall balance of Yin and Yang in the body.

This can lead to a range of health benefits, including improved digestion, increased energy, and a stronger immune system.

Chapter Five

The Importance of the Spleen and Stomach in TCM Nutrition

In Traditional Chinese Medicine (TCM), the spleen and stomach are considered to be the foundation of good health. The spleen and stomach are responsible for digestion and absorption of nutrients, as well as the transformation and transportation of food throughout the body. Below we will explore the importance of the spleen and stomach in TCM nutrition.

Functions of the Spleen and Stomach

The spleen and stomach are responsible for breaking down food and extracting nutrients. The spleen is responsible for transforming food into Qi (vital energy) and blood, while the stomach is responsible for digesting food and transporting it to the spleen.

In TCM, the spleen and stomach are also believed to play a role in maintaining the body's overall balance of Yin and Yang.

The Importance of Spleen Qi

In TCM, the concept of Qi is central to understanding the body's energy and vitality. The spleen is responsible for transforming food into Qi, which is then used to nourish the body and support bodily functions.

When the spleen is weak or imbalanced, Qi production is compromised, which can lead to a range of symptoms including fatigue, bloating, and poor digestion.

Eating for Spleen Health

In TCM nutrition, there are a number of dietary recommendations for supporting spleen health. Some of these include:

1. Eating warm, cooked foods: Raw or cold foods can weaken the spleen's ability to transform food into Qi. Eating warm, cooked foods can help to support spleen function.

2. Avoiding dampness: Dampness is believed to impair spleen function. Foods that are greasy or heavy can create dampness in the body, and should be avoided.

3. Eating at regular times: Eating at regular times can help to support the spleen's natural rhythms and improve digestion.

The Importance of Stomach Qi

In addition to the spleen, the stomach plays a critical role in TCM nutrition. The stomach is responsible for breaking down food and transporting it to the spleen for further processing.

When the stomach is weak or imbalanced, digestion can be compromised, leading to symptoms such as bloating, nausea, and poor appetite.

Eating for Stomach Health

In TCM nutrition, there are a number of dietary recommendations for supporting stomach health. Some of these include:

4. Eating slowly and mindfully: Eating slowly and mindfully can help to support the stomach's digestive function and prevent overeating.

5. Avoiding overeating: Overeating can put a strain on the stomach and impair its ability to digest food.

6. Eating easy-to-digest foods: Foods that are easy to digest, such as soups and stews, can help to support stomach function and improve digestion.

The role of the Spleen and Stomach in digestion

In Traditional Chinese Medicine (TCM), the spleen and stomach are considered to be the foundation of good health. The spleen and stomach are responsible for digestion and absorption of nutrients, as well as the transformation and transportation of food throughout the body. Below we will explore the role of the spleen and stomach in digestion in TCM nutrition.

The Role of the Spleen in Digestion

The spleen is responsible for transforming food into Qi (vital energy) and blood. It is also responsible for extracting nutrients from food and distributing them throughout the body.

The spleen is particularly important in the digestion of carbohydrates. Carbohydrates are broken down into glucose, which is then used by the body for energy. The spleen is responsible for transforming glucose into Qi, which is then used to nourish the body and support bodily functions.

The spleen also plays a role in the digestion of fats and proteins. These nutrients are broken down in the stomach and then transported to the spleen for further processing.

The Role of the Stomach in Digestion

The stomach is responsible for digesting food and transporting it to the spleen for further processing. It does this by using digestive juices, including hydrochloric acid and enzymes, to break down food into smaller particles.

The stomach is particularly important in the digestion of proteins. Proteins are broken down into amino acids, which are then used by the body for a variety of functions, including building muscle and repairing tissues.

The stomach also plays a role in the digestion of fats and carbohydrates. Fats are broken down into fatty acids, which are then used by the body for energy. Carbohydrates are broken down into glucose, which is also used by the body for energy.

The Importance of Spleen and Stomach Health

The health of the spleen and stomach is critical for proper digestion and nutrient absorption. When the spleen and stomach are functioning properly, nutrients are extracted from food and distributed throughout the body. However, when these organs are imbalanced or weakened, digestion can be compromised, leading to a range of symptoms including bloating, poor appetite, and fatigue.

Eating for Spleen and Stomach Health

In TCM nutrition, there are a number of dietary recommendations for supporting spleen and stomach health. Some of these include:

1. Eating warm, cooked foods: Raw or cold foods can weaken the spleen and stomach's ability to digest food. Eating warm, cooked foods can help to support digestive function.

2. Eating at regular times: Eating at regular times can help to support the spleen and stomach's natural rhythms and improve digestion.

3. Avoiding overeating: Overeating can put a strain on the spleen and stomach and impair their ability to digest food.

4. Eating easy-to-digest foods: Foods that are easy to digest, such as soups and stews, can help to support digestive function and improve nutrient absorption.

Supporting Spleen and Stomach function through diet

In Traditional Chinese Medicine (TCM), the spleen and stomach are considered to be the foundation of good health. The spleen and stomach are responsible for digestion and absorption of nutrients, as well as the transformation and transportation of food throughout the body. Below we will explore how to support spleen and stomach function through diet in TCM nutrition.

Eat Warm, Cooked Foods

In TCM, the spleen and stomach are believed to be weakened by cold or raw foods. Eating warm, cooked foods can help to support digestive function and strengthen the spleen and stomach. It is also recommended to avoid cold drinks and beverages, which can have a similar weakening effect.

Avoid Dampness

Dampness is believed to impair spleen function. Foods that are greasy or heavy can create dampness in the body, and should be avoided. It is also recommended to limit the consumption of dairy products, as they are believed to be damp-producing foods.

Eat at Regular Times

Eating at regular times can help to support the spleen and stomach's natural rhythms and improve digestion. It is recommended to eat three meals per day at roughly the same times each day, and to avoid skipping meals or eating irregularly.

Avoid Overeating

Overeating can put a strain on the spleen and stomach and impair their ability to digest food. It is recommended to eat until you are comfortably full, rather than overeating. It is also recommended to avoid eating too quickly, as this can also impair digestive function.

Eat Easy-to-Digest Foods

Foods that are easy to digest, such as soups and stews, can help to support digestive function and improve nutrient absorption. It is also recommended to chew food thoroughly, as this can help to improve digestion.

Use TCM Food Remedies

TCM food remedies are foods that have specific healing properties and are used to treat a range of health conditions. Some TCM food remedies that can be used to support spleen and stomach function include:

1. Ginger: Ginger is believed to stimulate the spleen and stomach and improve digestion. It can be added to soups, stews, and other dishes, or consumed as a tea.

2. Mung Beans: Mung beans are believed to be a cooling food that can help to clear dampness and support spleen function. They can be cooked and added to soups, stews, or salads.

3. Hawthorn Berries: Hawthorn berries are believed to improve digestion and regulate Qi flow. They can be consumed as a tea, or added to soups or stews.

Chapter Six

Dietary Guidelines for a Balanced TCM Diet

Traditional Chinese Medicine (TCM) has long recognized the connection between diet and health. TCM nutrition focuses on balancing the body's energy, or Qi, by consuming a balanced diet of foods that support the body's natural functions. Below we will explore dietary guidelines for a balanced TCM diet.

Eat a Variety of Foods

In TCM nutrition, it is recommended to eat a variety of foods to ensure that the body receives a range of nutrients. This includes consuming a variety of grains, vegetables, fruits, and protein sources. It is also recommended to eat foods of different colors, as different colors correspond to different organ systems in the body.

Eat According to the Seasons

In TCM nutrition, it is believed that the body's energy changes with the seasons. Eating according to the seasons can help to support the body's natural functions and maintain balance. For example, in the summer, it is recommended to eat cooling foods, such as watermelon and cucumber, while in the winter, it is recommended to eat warming foods, such as ginger and cinnamon.

Balance Yin and Yang

In TCM, balance is key to good health. The balance of Yin and Yang is particularly important in TCM nutrition. Foods are categorized as Yin or Yang based on their energetic properties. Yin foods are cooling and moistening, while Yang foods are warming and drying. It is recommended to balance Yin and Yang in the diet to maintain harmony and balance in the body.

Use Food Remedies

TCM food remedies are foods that have specific healing properties and are used to treat a range of health conditions. For example, ginger is believed to stimulate digestion and improve circulation, while turmeric is believed to have anti-inflammatory properties. Using food remedies can help to support the body's natural functions and maintain balance.

Avoid Processed Foods

In TCM nutrition, it is recommended to avoid processed foods, as they are believed to be damp-producing and can impair spleen function. Instead, it is recommended to eat fresh, whole foods that are prepared at home.

Eat Mindfully

In TCM, eating mindfully is important for maintaining balance and supporting digestive function. It is recommended to eat slowly and chew food thoroughly, as this can help to improve digestion. It is also recommended to eat in a relaxed and calm environment, as stress can impair digestive function.

Seek Guidance from a TCM Practitioner

Dietary recommendations in TCM are based on the individual's constitution and health needs. It is important to seek guidance from a qualified

TCM practitioner to determine the best diet for your individual needs and achieve optimal health and well-being.

Portion sizes and meal frequency

Portion sizes and meal frequency are important factors in maintaining a healthy diet in Traditional Chinese Medicine (TCM) nutrition. In TCM, it is believed that overeating or under-eating can disrupt the body's energy balance and lead to health problems. Below we will explore the importance of portion sizes and meal frequency in TCM nutrition.

Portion Sizes

In TCM nutrition, it is recommended to eat until you are comfortably full, rather than overeating. Overeating can put a strain on the digestive system, impair spleen function, and lead to weight gain. To avoid overeating, it is recommended to eat slowly and mindfully, chew food thoroughly, and take breaks during the meal to check for fullness.

In addition to avoiding overeating, it is important to ensure that portion sizes are appropriate for the individual's energy needs. TCM practitioners may use the concept of the "four divisions of the stomach" to determine appropriate portion sizes. This involves dividing the stomach into four parts, with one part each for food, liquid, air, and empty space. It is recommended to fill the food and liquid portions with appropriate amounts of food and beverage, leaving some space for air and empty space.

Meal Frequency

In TCM nutrition, it is recommended to eat three meals per day, with snacks as needed. Eating at regular times can help to support the body's natural rhythms and improve digestion. It is recommended to avoid skipping meals or eating irregularly, as this can disrupt the body's energy balance and impair digestive function.

In addition to eating regular meals, it is important to consider the timing of meals in relation to the body's energy patterns. In TCM, it is believed that the body's energy moves through different organ systems at different times of day. For example, the energy of the spleen and stomach is strongest in the morning, making breakfast an important meal. It is recommended to eat the largest meal of the day at lunchtime, when the body's energy is strongest, and to have a lighter meal in the evening, when the body's energy is weaker.

Balancing Yin and Yang

In TCM, balance is key to good health. This includes balancing Yin and Yang in the diet. Yin and Yang are opposing forces that need to be balanced to maintain harmony and balance in the body. Yin foods are cooling and moistening, while Yang foods are warming and drying. It is recommended to balance Yin and Yang in the diet to maintain harmony and balance in the body.

In relation to portion sizes and meal frequency, it is important to balance Yin and Yang in each meal. This means including appropriate amounts of Yin and Yang foods in each meal to maintain balance. For example, a meal that is high in Yang foods, such as meat and spices, may need to be balanced with Yin foods, such as vegetables and fruits.

Mindful Eating

In TCM nutrition, mindful eating is important for maintaining balance and supporting digestive function. It is recommended to eat in a relaxed and calm environment, as stress can impair digestive function. It is also recommended to eat slowly and chew food thoroughly, as this can help to improve digestion and nutrient absorption.

Combining foods for balance

In Traditional Chinese Medicine (TCM) nutrition, the way foods are combined can have a significant impact on the body's energy balance and overall health. By combining foods in a balanced way, it is possible to support the body's natural functions and maintain optimal health and well-being. Below we will explore the importance of combining foods for balance in TCM nutrition.

The Five Flavors

1. In TCM, foods are categorized by their energetic properties, including the five flavors: sweet, sour, bitter, pungent, and salty. Each flavor is associated with a different organ system in the body and has specific energetic properties that can impact the body's energy balance. For example, sweet foods are associated with the spleen and stomach and are nourishing and moistening, while bitter foods are associated with the heart and small intestine and are drying and cooling.

To balance the body's energy, it is important to include all five flavors in the diet and combine them in a balanced way. This means including appropriate amounts of each flavor in each meal to maintain balance.

The Five Elements

2. In addition to the five flavors, foods are also categorized by the five elements: wood, fire, earth, metal, and water. Each element is associated with a different organ system in the body and has specific energetic properties that can impact the body's energy balance. For example, the wood element is associated with the liver and gallbladder and is associated with growth

and expansion, while the metal element is associated with the lungs and large intestine and is associated with contraction and elimination.

To balance the body's energy, it is important to include a variety of foods from each element in the diet and combine them in a balanced way. This means including appropriate amounts of each element in each meal to maintain balance.

Food Combining Rules

In TCM nutrition, there are specific rules for combining foods to maintain balance. These rules include:

Eating grains and vegetables together, as grains are Yang and vegetables are Yin, and the combination helps to balance Yin and Yang.

Eating fruits alone or on an empty stomach, as fruits are Yin and can impair digestion when combined with Yang foods.

Avoiding combining animal protein with grains or starchy vegetables, as this can impair digestion and lead to dampness in the body.

Combining protein with non-starchy vegetables, as this can help to balance Yin and Yang and support digestion.

Combining grains with legumes or nuts, as this can help to balance Yin and Yang and provide a complete protein source.

Individualized Recommendations

In TCM nutrition, dietary recommendations are based on the individual's constitution and health needs. This means that food combining recommendations may vary from person to person. For example, a person with a weak digestive system may need to avoid certain food combinations, while a person with a strong digestive system may be able to tolerate them.

It is important to consult with a qualified TCM practitioner to determine the best food combining recommendations for your individual needs and achieve optimal health and well-being.

Chapter Seven

TCM Nutrition for Specific Body Constitutions

In Traditional Chinese Medicine (TCM) nutrition, dietary recommendations are based on the individual's body constitution. Each person has a unique body constitution that is determined by a combination of genetic, environmental, and lifestyle factors. By understanding an individual's body constitution, it is possible to tailor dietary recommendations to their specific needs and achieve optimal health and well-being. Below we will explore TCM nutrition for specific body constitutions.

The Five Body Constitutions

1. In TCM, there are five body constitutions: Wood, Fire, Earth, Metal, and Water. Each body constitution is associated with specific organs and energy patterns in the body, as well as specific dietary recommendations.

2. Wood: The Wood constitution is associated with the liver and gallbladder and is characterized by a tendency towards anger and frustration. Dietary recommendations for the Wood constitution include a focus on bitter and sour flavors, as well as foods that promote the flow of Qi, such as cruciferous vegetables, citrus fruits, and ginger.

3. Fire: The Fire constitution is associated with the heart and small intestine and is characterized by a tendency towards excitability and anxiety. Dietary recommendations for the Fire constitution include a focus on bitter and cooling foods, such as bitter greens, cucumbers, and celery.

4. Earth: The Earth constitution is associated with the spleen and stomach and is characterized by a tendency towards worry and overthinking. Dietary recommendations for the Earth constitution include a focus on sweet and nourishing foods, such as whole grains, root vegetables, and legumes.

5. Metal: The Metal constitution is associated with the lungs and large intestine and is characterized by a tendency towards perfectionism and rigidity. Dietary recommendations for the Metal constitution include a focus on pungent and warming foods, such as onions, garlic, and ginger, as well as foods that promote the flow of Qi and moisten the lungs, such as pears and honey.

6. Water: The Water constitution is associated with the kidneys and bladder and is characterized by a tendency towards fear and insecurity. Dietary recommendations for the Water constitution include a focus on salty and warming foods, such as seaweed, miso soup, and fish.

Yin and Yang Imbalances

In addition to the five body constitutions, TCM also considers imbalances in Yin and Yang energy in the body. Yin and Yang are opposing forces that need to be balanced to maintain harmony and balance in the body. Yin energy is associated with cooling, moistening, and calming, while Yang energy is associated with warming, drying, and stimulating.

If an individual has an imbalance of Yin or Yang energy in the body, dietary recommendations may be adjusted to promote balance. For example, if an individual has an excess of Yang energy, they may be advised to eat more Yin foods, such as cooling fruits and vegetables, and avoid spicy or warming foods.

Mindful Eating

In TCM nutrition, mindful eating is important for maintaining balance and supporting digestive function. It is recommended to eat in a relaxed and calm environment, as stress can impair digestive function. It is also recommended to eat slowly and chew food thoroughly, as this can help to improve digestion and nutrient absorption.

Identifying your body constitution

In Traditional Chinese Medicine (TCM), identifying your body constitution is an important step in understanding your individual health needs and tailoring dietary recommendations to your unique needs. Each person has a unique body constitution that is determined by a combination of genetic, environmental, and lifestyle factors. By identifying your body constitution, it is possible to make dietary adjustments to support optimal health and well-being. Below we will explore how to identify your body constitution in TCM.

Consult with a TCM Practitioner

The most accurate way to identify your body constitution in TCM is to consult with a qualified TCM practitioner. A TCM practitioner can assess your health history, physical symptoms, and pulse and tongue diagnosis to determine your body constitution and make dietary recommendations based on your unique needs.

Self-Assessment

While consulting with a TCM practitioner is the most accurate way to identify your body constitution, there are also self-assessment tools that can provide some insight into your constitution. These tools can be used as a starting point to guide your dietary choices.

1. Symptoms: Consider any physical symptoms you experience on a regular basis, such as digestive issues, headaches, or muscle tension. These symptoms can provide insight into your body constitution and help guide your dietary choices.

2. Personality: Consider your personality traits and tendencies. Are you easily angered or frustrated? Do you tend to worry or overthink? These traits can provide insight into your body constitution and help guide your dietary choices.

3. Food preferences: Consider your food preferences. Do you tend to crave sweet foods or salty foods? These preferences can provide insight into your body constitution and help guide your dietary choices.

Body Constitution Types

In TCM, there are five body constitution types: Wood, Fire, Earth, Metal, and Water. Each body constitution type is associated with specific organs and energy patterns in the body, as well as specific dietary recommendations. Here is a brief overview of each body constitution type:

4. Wood: The Wood constitution is associated with the liver and gallbladder and is characterized by a tendency towards anger and frustration.

5. Fire: The Fire constitution is associated with the heart and small intestine and is characterized by a tendency towards excitability and anxiety.

6. Earth: The Earth constitution is associated with the spleen and stomach and is characterized by a tendency towards worry and overthinking.

7. Metal: The Metal constitution is associated with the lungs and large intestine and is characterized by a tendency towards perfectionism and rigidity.

8. Water: The Water constitution is associated with the kidneys and bladder and is characterized by a tendency towards fear and insecurity.

Balancing Your Body Constitution

Once you have identified your body constitution, you can make dietary adjustments to support optimal health and well-being. This may include incorporating specific flavors, elements, and food combining rules into your diet to maintain balance. It is important to consult with a qualified TCM practitioner to determine the best dietary recommendations for your individual needs.

Tailoring your diet to your constitution

In Traditional Chinese Medicine (TCM) nutrition, tailoring your diet to your constitution is essential for achieving optimal health and well-being. Each person has a unique body constitution that is determined by a combination of genetic, environmental, and lifestyle factors. By understanding your body constitution, it is possible to tailor your diet to your unique needs and achieve balance in the body. Below we will explore how to tailor your diet to your constitution in TCM.

Identify Your Body Constitution

The first step in tailoring your diet to your constitution is to identify your body constitution. This can be done through self-assessment or by consulting with a qualified TCM practitioner. By identifying your body constitution, you can make dietary adjustments to support your unique needs and promote optimal health and well-being.

Choose Foods According to Your Body Constitution

In TCM, each body constitution is associated with specific flavors, elements, and food groups. By incorporating these into your diet, you can support your body constitution and promote balance in the body. Here are some general guidelines for each body constitution:

1. Wood: The Wood constitution is associated with the liver and gallbladder and is characterized by a tendency towards anger and frustration. Dietary recommendations for the Wood constitution include a focus on bitter and sour flavors, as well as foods that promote the flow of Qi, such as cruciferous vegetables, citrus fruits, and ginger.

2. Fire: The Fire constitution is associated with the heart and small intestine and is characterized by a tendency towards excitability and anxiety. Dietary recommendations for the Fire constitution include a focus on bitter and cooling foods, such as bitter greens, cucumbers, and celery.

3. Earth: The Earth constitution is associated with the spleen and stomach and is characterized by a tendency towards worry and overthinking. Dietary recommendations for the Earth constitution include a focus on sweet and nourishing foods, such as whole grains, root vegetables, and legumes.

4. Metal: The Metal constitution is associated with the lungs and large intestine and is characterized by a tendency towards perfectionism and rigidity. Dietary recommendations for the Metal constitution include a focus on pungent and warming foods, such as onions, garlic, and ginger, as well as foods that promote the flow of Qi and moisten the lungs, such as pears and honey.

5. Water: The Water constitution is associated with the kidneys and bladder and is characterized by a tendency towards fear and insecurity. Dietary recommendations for the Water constitution include a focus on salty and warming foods, such as seaweed, miso soup, and fish.

Consider the Energetic Properties of Foods

In TCM, the energetic properties of foods are also important to consider when tailoring your diet to your constitution. Foods are classified as hot, warm, neutral, cool, or cold, depending on their energetic properties. By choosing foods that balance your constitution, you can promote optimal health and well-being. Here are some general guidelines for choosing foods according to their energetic properties:

6. Hot foods: Hot foods are warming and can help promote circulation and energy flow in the body. They are recommended for individuals with a cold constitution or those who live in a cold environment.

7. Warm foods: Warm foods are nourishing and can help promote digestion and nutrient absorption. They are recommended for individuals with a weak constitution or those who are recovering from illness.

8. Neutral foods: Neutral foods have a balancing effect on the body and can help maintain overall health and well-being. They are recommended for individuals with a balanced constitution.

9. Cool foods: Cool foods are cooling and can help reduce inflammation and heat in the body. They are recommended for individuals with a hot constitution or those who live in a hot environment.

10. Cold foods: Cold foods are cooling and can help reduce inflammation and heat in the body. They are

Chapter Eight

TCM Nutrition for Seasonal Health

In Traditional Chinese Medicine (TCM) nutrition, seasonal changes are considered an important factor in maintaining optimal health and well-being. Each season has its unique energy and elemental qualities, and by adjusting our diet to support these changes, we can promote balance in the body and prevent illness. Below we will explore TCM nutrition for seasonal health.

Spring

Spring is associated with the Wood element and the liver and gallbladder organs. In TCM, spring is a time of renewal and growth, and it is important to support the liver in this process. Foods that are recommended for spring include bitter greens, such as dandelion and arugula, as well as sprouts and young plants. It is also recommended to avoid heavy and greasy foods, such as fried foods and dairy, as they can burden the liver.

Summer

Summer is associated with the Fire element and the heart and small intestine organs. In TCM, summer is a time of heat and energy, and it is important to stay hydrated and cool. Foods that are recommended for summer include cooling and hydrating fruits and vegetables, such as watermelon, cucumber, and mint. It is also recommended to avoid excessive amounts of spicy or greasy foods, as they can contribute to heat in the body.

Late Summer

Late summer is associated with the Earth element and the spleen and stomach organs. In TCM, late summer is a time of transformation and transition, and it is important to support the digestive system. Foods that are recommended for late summer include sweet and nourishing foods, such as root vegetables, whole grains, and legumes. It is also recommended to avoid raw and cold foods, as they can impair digestion.

Fall

Fall is associated with the Metal element and the lungs and large intestine organs. In TCM, fall is a time of letting go and releasing, and it is important to support the lungs in this process. Foods that are recommended for fall include pungent and warming foods, such as onions, garlic, and ginger, as well as foods that moisten the lungs, such as pears and honey. It is also recommended to avoid excessive amounts of raw and cold foods, as they can impair the lungs.

Winter

Winter is associated with the Water element and the kidneys and bladder organs. In TCM, winter is a time of rest and conservation, and it is important to support the kidneys in this process. Foods that are recommended for winter include warming and nourishing foods, such as soups and stews, as well as root vegetables and animal protein. It is also recommended to avoid excessive amounts of raw and cold foods, as they can impair kidney function.

General Dietary Recommendations

In addition to seasonal adjustments, there are also general dietary recommendations in TCM that can support overall health and well-being. These include:

1. Eating a variety of whole foods: TCM emphasizes the importance of eating a variety of whole foods to support overall health and well-being.

2. Eating mindfully: TCM also emphasizes the importance of eating mindfully, taking time to chew food thoroughly and savoring the flavors.

3. Avoiding processed and refined foods: TCM recommends avoiding processed and refined foods, as they can disrupt the body's natural balance.

4. Drinking warm or room temperature liquids: TCM recommends drinking warm or room temperature liquids, as cold liquids can impair digestion.

5. Eating in moderation: TCM also recommends eating in moderation, avoiding excesses in any one food group.

Eating according to the seasons

In traditional Chinese medicine (TCM), diet and nutrition play a crucial role in promoting health and preventing illness. TCM emphasizes the importance of eating according to the seasons, which means that the foods we consume should be chosen based on the season and the energy of that season. By eating seasonally, we can help maintain balance in the body and promote optimal health. Below we will explore the benefits of eating according to the seasons in TCM nutrition.

Spring

Spring is a time of renewal and growth. It is associated with the Wood element and the liver and gallbladder organs. In TCM, spring is the perfect time to detoxify the body and support liver function. It is recommended to eat fresh and light foods, such as leafy greens, sprouts, and young plants. These foods can help nourish the liver and promote healthy digestion. It is also recommended to avoid heavy and greasy foods, as they can burden the liver and disrupt its function.

Summer

Summer is a time of heat and energy. It is associated with the Fire element and the heart and small intestine organs. In TCM, summer is the perfect time to stay hydrated and cool. It is recommended to eat cooling and hydrating foods, such as watermelon, cucumber, and mint. These foods can help regulate body temperature and support healthy digestion. It is also recommended to avoid excessive amounts of spicy or greasy foods, as they can contribute to heat in the body.

Late Summer

Late summer is associated with the Earth element and the spleen and stomach organs. In TCM, late summer is a time of transformation and transition. It is recommended to eat sweet and nourishing foods, such as root vegetables, whole grains, and legumes. These foods can help support healthy digestion and strengthen the spleen and stomach. It is also recommended to avoid raw and cold foods, as they can impair digestion.

Fall

Fall is a time of letting go and releasing. It is associated with the Metal element and the lungs and large intestine organs. In TCM, fall is the perfect time to support lung function and promote healthy immune function. It is recommended to eat pungent and warming foods, such as onions, garlic, and ginger, as well as foods that moisten the lungs, such as pears and honey. These foods can help support healthy lung function and promote healthy immune function. It is also recommended to avoid excessive amounts of raw and cold foods, as they can impair lung function.

Winter

Winter is a time of rest and conservation. It is associated with the Water element and the kidneys and bladder organs. In TCM, winter is the perfect time to support kidney function and promote healthy energy levels. It is recommended to eat warming and nourishing foods, such as soups and stews, as well as root vegetables and animal protein. These foods can help support healthy kidney function and promote healthy energy levels. It is also recommended to avoid excessive amounts of raw and cold foods, as they can impair kidney function.

General Dietary Recommendations

In addition to eating seasonally, there are also general dietary recommendations in TCM that can support overall health and well-being. These include:

1. Eating a variety of whole foods: TCM emphasizes the importance of eating a variety of whole foods to support overall health and well-being.

2. Eating mindfully: TCM also emphasizes the importance of eating mindfully, taking time to chew food thoroughly and savoring the flavors.

3. Avoiding processed and refined foods: TCM recommends avoiding processed and refined foods, as they can disrupt the body's natural balance.

4. Drinking warm or room temperature liquids: TCM recommends drinking warm or room temperature liquids, as cold liquids can impair digestion.

Eating in

Seasonal foods and their benefits

In traditional Chinese medicine (TCM), diet and nutrition play a crucial role in promoting health and preventing illness. Eating seasonally is an important aspect of TCM nutrition, as it helps to maintain balance in the body and promote optimal health. Each season offers a unique variety of foods that are in tune with the energy of that season. Below we will explore the benefits of seasonal foods in TCM nutrition.

Spring Foods

Spring is a time of renewal and growth. It is associated with the Wood element and the liver and gallbladder organs. In TCM, spring is the perfect time to detoxify the body and support liver function. Some spring foods that are recommended in TCM include:

1. Leafy greens: Leafy greens are a great source of vitamins and minerals, and they help to support healthy liver function.

2. Sprouts: Sprouts are nutrient-dense and easy to digest, making them a great choice for spring.

3. Young plants: Young plants, such as asparagus and dandelion greens, are full of vitamins and minerals and can help support healthy digestion.

Summer Foods

Summer is a time of heat and energy. It is associated with the Fire element and the heart and small intestine organs. In TCM, summer is the perfect time to stay hydrated and cool. Some summer foods that are recommended in TCM include:

4. Watermelon: Watermelon is hydrating and cooling, making it a great choice for summer.

5. Cucumber: Cucumbers are also hydrating and cooling, and they help to support healthy digestion.

6. Mint: Mint is cooling and refreshing, making it a great addition to summer drinks and dishes.

Late Summer Foods

Late summer is associated with the Earth element and the spleen and stomach organs. In TCM, late summer is a time of transformation and transition. Some late summer foods that are recommended in TCM include:

7. Root vegetables: Root vegetables, such as sweet potatoes and carrots, are grounding and nourishing, and they help to support healthy digestion.

8. Whole grains: Whole grains, such as brown rice and quinoa, are also grounding and nourishing, and they help to support healthy digestion.

9. Legumes: Legumes, such as lentils and beans, are a great source of protein and fiber, and they help to support healthy digestion.

Fall Foods

Fall is a time of letting go and releasing. It is associated with the Metal element and the lungs and large intestine organs. In TCM, fall is the perfect time to support lung function and promote healthy immune function. Some fall foods that are recommended in TCM include:

10. Pears: Pears are a great source of fiber and help to moisten the lungs, making them a great choice for fall.

11. Honey: Honey is also moistening and can help to soothe the throat and promote healthy immune function.

12. Onions and garlic: Onions and garlic are pungent and warming, making them a great addition to fall dishes.

Winter Foods

Winter is a time of rest and conservation. It is associated with the Water element and the kidneys and bladder organs. In TCM, winter is the perfect time to support kidney function and promote healthy energy levels. Some winter foods that are recommended in TCM include:

13. Root vegetables: Root vegetables, such as turnips and parsnips, are grounding and nourishing, and they help to support healthy kidney function.

14. Animal protein: Animal protein, such as beef and chicken, is warming and nourishing, making it a great choice for winter.

15. Soups and stews: Soups and stews are warming and easy to digest, making them a great choice for winter.

Chapter Nine

Food Therapy for Common Health Conditions

In traditional Chinese medicine (TCM), food therapy is used to prevent and treat common health conditions. TCM nutrition focuses on the energetic properties of foods and how they interact with the body. By choosing the right foods and cooking them in the right way, we can promote health and prevent disease. Below we will explore food therapy for common health conditions.

Digestive Issues

Digestive issues, such as bloating, gas, and constipation, are common in TCM. In TCM, digestion is controlled by the Spleen and Stomach organs. To promote healthy digestion, it is important to eat foods that are easy to digest and that support the Spleen and Stomach. Some foods that are recommended for digestive issues in TCM include:

1. Ginger: Ginger is warming and helps to stimulate digestion. It can be added to soups, stews, and teas.

2. Rice porridge: Rice porridge is easy to digest and can help to soothe the digestive system.

3. Cooked vegetables: Cooked vegetables, such as carrots, zucchini, and pumpkin, are easy to digest and can help to support the Spleen and Stomach.

Respiratory Issues

Respiratory issues, such as coughs, colds, and allergies, are common in TCM. In TCM, the lungs are responsible for breathing and the immune system. To promote healthy respiratory function, it is important to eat foods that are moistening and support the lungs. Some foods that are recommended for respiratory issues in TCM include:

4. Pears: Pears are moistening and can help to soothe a dry cough.

5. Honey: Honey is also moistening and can help to soothe a sore throat.

6. Mushrooms: Mushrooms, such as shiitake and reishi, can help to boost the immune system and support healthy respiratory function.

Stress and Anxiety

Stress and anxiety are common in TCM. In TCM, stress and anxiety are caused by a lack of Qi (energy) in the body. To promote healthy Qi flow and reduce stress and anxiety, it is important to eat foods that are nourishing and support the Heart and Kidney organs. Some foods that are recommended for stress and anxiety in TCM include:

7. Oats: Oats are nourishing and can help to soothe the nervous system.

8. Black beans: Black beans are nourishing and can help to support healthy Kidney function.

9. Dark leafy greens: Dark leafy greens, such as spinach and kale, are rich in vitamins and minerals and can help to support the Heart and Kidney organs.

Menstrual Issues

Menstrual issues, such as cramps and irregular periods, are common in TCM. In TCM, menstrual issues are caused by a lack of Qi and Blood flow in the body. To promote healthy Qi and Blood flow and reduce menstrual issues, it is important to eat foods that are nourishing and support the Spleen and Liver organs. Some foods that are recommended for menstrual issues in TCM include:

10. Dates: Dates are nourishing and can help to promote healthy Blood flow.

11. Dark leafy greens: Dark leafy greens are rich in iron and can help to support healthy Blood flow.

12. Ginger tea: Ginger tea can help to stimulate Qi and Blood flow and reduce menstrual cramps.

Insomnia

Insomnia is common in TCM. In TCM, insomnia is caused by a lack of Yin and Blood in the body. To promote healthy Yin and Blood flow and reduce insomnia, it is important to eat foods that are nourishing and support the Heart and Kidney organs. Some foods that are recommended for insomnia in TCM include:

Wal

TCM nutrition for digestive issues

In traditional Chinese medicine (TCM), the digestive system is considered to be the foundation of good health. A healthy digestive system is essential for the proper absorption and distribution of nutrients throughout the body. When the digestive system is not functioning properly, it can lead to a variety of health issues, such as bloating, gas, and constipation. TCM nutrition can play an important role in promoting healthy digestion and treating digestive issues.

In TCM, digestion is controlled by the Spleen and Stomach organs. The Spleen is responsible for transforming food into Qi (energy) and Blood, while the Stomach is responsible for breaking down food and absorbing nutrients. When the Spleen and Stomach are not functioning properly, it can lead to digestive issues.

To promote healthy digestion and treat digestive issues, TCM nutrition focuses on eating foods that are easy to digest and that support the Spleen and Stomach. Some foods that are recommended for digestive issues in TCM include:

Ginger

Ginger is a warming herb that helps to stimulate digestion. It can be added to soups, stews, and teas. Ginger also has anti-inflammatory properties that can help to reduce inflammation in the digestive system.

Rice porridge

Rice porridge is a traditional TCM remedy for digestive issues. It is easy to digest and can help to soothe the digestive system. Rice porridge can be made with white rice or brown rice and can be flavored with ginger, cinnamon, or honey.

Cooked vegetables

Cooked vegetables are easy to digest and can help to support the Spleen and Stomach. Some vegetables that are recommended for digestive issues in TCM include carrots, zucchini, pumpkin, and winter squash. These vegetables can be cooked in soups, stews, or steamed and served with a light seasoning.

Bone broth

Bone broth is a nourishing food that is rich in nutrients and easy to digest. It is made by simmering bones, such as chicken or beef bones, for several hours with vegetables and herbs. Bone broth can be consumed on its own or used as a base for soups and stews.

Fermented foods

Fermented foods, such as sauerkraut, kimchi, and miso, are rich in probiotics that can help to promote healthy gut bacteria. Probiotics can help to improve digestion and reduce digestive issues, such as bloating and gas.

Herbal teas

Herbal teas, such as peppermint, chamomile, and fennel, can help to soothe the digestive system and reduce digestive issues. Peppermint tea can help to relieve bloating and gas, while chamomile tea can help to reduce inflammation in the digestive system.

In addition to eating foods that support healthy digestion, TCM nutrition also recommends practicing mindful eating habits. This includes eating slowly, chewing food thoroughly, and avoiding overeating. It is also recommended to avoid eating raw, cold, or greasy foods, as these can be difficult to digest and can exacerbate digestive issues.

TCM nutrition for immune support

In traditional Chinese medicine (TCM), the immune system is closely connected to the digestive system. Good digestion is essential for a strong immune system, as it allows the body to properly absorb and utilize nutrients that support immune function. TCM nutrition can play an important role in supporting the immune system and helping to prevent illness.

TCM nutrition recommends eating a balanced diet that includes a variety of whole, nutrient-dense foods. Some foods that are particularly beneficial for immune support include:

Shiitake mushrooms

Shiitake mushrooms are rich in beta-glucans, which are complex sugars that can stimulate the immune system. They also contain polysaccharides, which can help to boost immune function and reduce inflammation in the body.

Garlic

Garlic has been used for centuries in TCM to support the immune system. It contains compounds, such as allicin and sulfur, that have antibacterial and antiviral properties. Garlic can also help to stimulate the production of white blood cells, which are an important part of the immune system.

Ginger

Ginger is a warming herb that can help to improve circulation and boost immune function. It also has anti-inflammatory properties that can help to reduce inflammation in the body.

Bone broth

Bone broth is a nutrient-dense food that can help to support the immune system. It is rich in amino acids, collagen, and minerals that are essential for immune function. Bone broth can also help to reduce inflammation in the body, which can help to support overall health.

Turmeric

Turmeric is a powerful anti-inflammatory herb that can help to support immune function. It contains a compound called curcumin, which has been shown to have antimicrobial and antiviral properties. Turmeric can be added to soups, stews, and teas for a boost of immune support.

Green leafy vegetables

Green leafy vegetables, such as spinach, kale, and collard greens, are rich in nutrients that are essential for immune function. They are also rich in antioxidants, which can help to reduce inflammation in the body.

In addition to eating foods that support immune function, TCM nutrition also recommends practicing good eating habits that support overall health. This includes eating a variety of whole, nutrient-dense foods, avoiding processed foods and refined sugars, and staying hydrated.

TCM also recommends avoiding foods that can weaken the immune system, such as:

Sugar

Consuming too much sugar can weaken the immune system and make the body more susceptible to illness. This is because sugar can interfere with the function of white blood cells, which are an important part of the immune system.

Alcohol

Drinking excessive amounts of alcohol can weaken the immune system and increase the risk of infections. This is because alcohol can interfere with the function of white blood cells and other immune cells.

Processed foods

Processed foods are often high in salt, sugar, and unhealthy fats, which can weaken the immune system and increase the risk of illness. They are also low in nutrients that are essential for immune function.

Chapter Ten

Herbal Remedies in TCM Nutrition

Herbal remedies have been a cornerstone of traditional Chinese medicine (TCM) for centuries. In TCM nutrition, herbs are often used in combination with whole foods to support overall health and well-being. TCM practitioners use herbs to address specific health concerns and to promote balance and harmony in the body.

Herbs in TCM are classified according to their energetic properties, taste, and actions in the body. Some of the most commonly used herbs in TCM nutrition include:

Ginseng

Ginseng is one of the most well-known herbs in TCM. It is a powerful adaptogen, which means that it can help the body adapt to stress and promote overall balance and harmony. Ginseng is also believed to help improve cognitive function, boost energy, and support the immune system.

Astragalus

Astragalus is another adaptogenic herb that is commonly used in TCM. It is believed to help support the immune system and improve overall health and well-being. Astragalus is often used in combination with other herbs to support digestive function and improve energy levels.

Licorice root

Licorice root is a sweet-tasting herb that is often used in TCM to support digestive function and soothe the throat and respiratory system. It is also believed to help support the immune system and improve overall health and well-being.

Turmeric

Turmeric is a bright yellow spice that is commonly used in TCM to support digestive function and reduce inflammation in the body. It contains a compound called curcumin, which has been shown to have powerful antioxidant and anti-inflammatory properties.

Reishi mushroom

Reishi mushroom is a powerful adaptogen that is commonly used in TCM to support immune function and promote overall health and well-being. It is also believed to help improve cognitive function and reduce inflammation in the body.

Schisandra

Schisandra is a sour-tasting herb that is often used in TCM to support liver function and improve overall health and well-being. It is also believed to help improve cognitive function, reduce inflammation, and support the immune system.

Hawthorn berry

Hawthorn berry is a sweet-tasting herb that is often used in TCM to support cardiovascular function and improve overall health and well-being. It is also believed to have antioxidant properties and help improve digestive function.

In addition to using herbs in TCM nutrition, TCM practitioners also use herbal remedies to address specific health concerns. For example, some common herbal remedies in TCM include:

Echinacea

Echinacea is a popular herbal remedy that is commonly used to support immune function and reduce the duration and severity of colds and other respiratory infections.

Milk thistle

Milk thistle is a common herbal remedy that is used to support liver function and promote detoxification in the body. It is also believed to have antioxidant properties and may help to reduce inflammation in the body.

Saw palmetto

Saw palmetto is a popular herbal remedy that is used to support prostate health in men. It is believed to help reduce inflammation in the prostate gland and improve urinary function.

Valerian root

Valerian root is a commonly used herbal remedy that is used to promote relaxation and improve sleep quality. It is believed to have sedative properties that can help to calm the nervous system and reduce stress and anxiety.

St. John's Wort

St. John's Wort is a popular herbal remedy that is used to support mood and emotional well-being. It is believed to help reduce symptoms of mild to moderate depression and anxiety.

It is important to note that herbal remedies should always be used under the guidance of a qualified TCM practitioner. Some herbs can interact with medications or have side effects,

Common TCM herbs and their benefits

Traditional Chinese medicine (TCM) is a holistic approach to healthcare that has been practiced for thousands of years. Herbs are an essential component of TCM, and they are used to address a wide range of health concerns. Here are some common TCM herbs and their benefits:

Dang Gui (Angelica sinensis)

Dang Gui is a popular TCM herb that is often used to support women's health. It is believed to help regulate menstrual cycles and reduce symptoms of premenstrual syndrome (PMS). Dang Gui is also used to support digestive function, improve circulation, and promote overall health and well-being.

Bai Zhu (Atractylodes macrocephala)

Bai Zhu is a commonly used TCM herb that is believed to help support digestive function and improve energy levels. It is often used in combination with other herbs to support digestive health and reduce inflammation in the body.

Huang Qi (Astragalus membranaceus)

Huang Qi is a popular TCM herb that is often used to support immune function and improve overall health and well-being. It is believed to help boost energy levels, reduce inflammation, and improve cardiovascular function.

Gan Cao (Licorice root)

Gan Cao is a sweet-tasting herb that is often used in TCM to support digestive function and soothe the throat and respiratory system. It is also believed to help support the immune system and improve overall health and well-being.

Chuan Xiong (Ligusticum chuanxiong)

Chuan Xiong is a TCM herb that is often used to support women's health. It is believed to help regulate menstrual cycles and reduce symptoms of PMS. Chuan Xiong is also used to support cardiovascular function and improve blood flow to the brain.

Ren Shen (Ginseng)

Ren Shen is one of the most well-known TCM herbs. It is a powerful adaptogen that is believed to help the body adapt to stress and promote overall balance and harmony. Ginseng is also believed to help improve cognitive function, boost energy, and support the immune system.

Shan Zha (Hawthorn berry)

Shan Zha is a sweet-tasting herb that is often used in TCM to support cardiovascular function and improve overall health and well-being. It is also believed to have antioxidant properties and help improve digestive function.

Shi Gao (Gypsum)

Shi Gao is a TCM herb that is often used to reduce inflammation and fever in the body. It is believed to have a cooling effect on the body and can be useful in treating conditions such as sore throat, cough, and bronchitis.

He Shou Wu (Polygonum multiflorum)

He Shou Wu is a TCM herb that is often used to support the liver and kidney function. It is believed to help improve energy levels, reduce inflammation, and promote overall health and well-being.

Bai Shao (White peony root)

Bai Shao is a TCM herb that is often used to support women's health. It is believed to help regulate menstrual cycles and reduce symptoms of PMS. Bai Shao is also used to support digestive function and reduce inflammation in the body.

In addition to these commonly used TCM herbs, there are many other herbs that are used in TCM to address specific health concerns. It is important to note that herbs should always be used under the guidance of a qualified TCM practitioner, as some herbs can interact with medications or have side effects.

Incorporating herbs into your diet

Herbs are an integral part of traditional Chinese medicine (TCM) and have been used for thousands of years to promote health and well-being. Incorporating herbs into your diet is a great way to support your body's natural healing processes and improve your overall health. Here are some tips for incorporating herbs into your diet:

Start with simple recipes

If you are new to using herbs in your diet, it is best to start with simple recipes that use just a few herbs. For example, you could try adding ginger to your morning smoothie or brewing a cup of chamomile tea before bed. As you become more comfortable using herbs, you can start experimenting with more complex recipes and blends.

Use fresh herbs whenever possible

Fresh herbs are often more potent and flavorful than dried herbs, so it is best to use fresh herbs whenever possible. You can grow your own herbs at home or purchase fresh herbs from a local farmer's market or health food store.

Experiment with different flavors

One of the benefits of incorporating herbs into your diet is that they can add a variety of flavors to your meals. For example, rosemary adds a savory, earthy flavor to roasted vegetables, while mint adds a refreshing, cooling flavor to salads and smoothies. Experiment with different herbs to find the flavors that you enjoy the most.

Use herbs to replace unhealthy ingredients

Many herbs have medicinal properties that can help support your health. For example, garlic has been shown to have antibacterial and antiviral properties, while turmeric has anti-inflammatory properties. Instead of using unhealthy ingredients like processed sugar or salt, try using herbs like garlic and turmeric to add flavor to your meals.

Consider taking herbal supplements

In addition to incorporating herbs into your diet, you may also want to consider taking herbal supplements. TCM practitioners often recommend specific herbal formulas to address specific health concerns. These formulas can be taken in capsule or powder form and are designed to support your body's natural healing processes.

Work with a qualified TCM practitioner

If you are interested in incorporating herbs into your diet or taking herbal supplements, it is important to work with a qualified TCM practitioner.

They can help you determine which herbs are right for you and how to use them safely and effectively. They can also help you address specific health concerns using TCM principles and practices.

Chapter Eleven

TCM Nutritional Approaches to Weight Management

Traditional Chinese Medicine (TCM) offers a holistic approach to weight management that considers not only what we eat, but how and when we eat, as well as the emotional and energetic factors that may contribute to weight gain. Here are some TCM nutritional approaches to weight management:

Eating for your body constitution

According to TCM principles, each person has a unique body constitution that determines their physical and emotional characteristics, as well as their susceptibility to certain health conditions. By eating according to your body constitution, you can promote balance and harmony within your body, which can support healthy weight management. For example, if you have a "damp" constitution, you may be more prone to weight gain and digestive issues, so you may need to avoid damp-producing foods like dairy and processed foods and focus on warming, drying foods like ginger and whole grains.

Balancing Yin and Yang

Another key principle of TCM is the concept of Yin and Yang, which represent opposing yet complementary forces within the body. In terms of nutrition, Yin foods are cooling and nourishing, while Yang foods are warming and invigorating. To support healthy weight management, it is important to balance these two energies. For example, if you tend to eat a lot of Yang foods like spicy or fried foods, you may need to balance it out with more Yin foods like leafy greens and fruits.

Mindful eating

TCM also emphasizes the importance of mindful eating, which means paying attention to your body's hunger and fullness cues, as well as the quality and quantity of the food you are eating. By eating slowly, savoring each bite, and focusing on the flavors and textures of your food, you can better regulate your appetite and avoid overeating.

Meal timing

In TCM, meal timing is also considered important for healthy digestion and weight management. It is recommended to eat a light breakfast to kickstart your metabolism, a moderate lunch to sustain your energy throughout the day, and a small dinner to avoid overloading your digestive system at night. It is also recommended to avoid eating late at night, as this can disrupt your sleep and lead to weight gain.

Herbal remedies

In addition to dietary approaches, TCM also uses herbal remedies to support healthy weight management. For example, herbs like cinnamon and ginger can help regulate blood sugar and boost metabolism, while bitter herbs like dandelion and burdock can support liver and digestive function.

Acupuncture

Acupuncture is another TCM modality that can be helpful for weight management. By targeting specific acupressure points on the body, acupuncture can help regulate appetite, reduce cravings, and support healthy digestion and metabolism.

The TCM perspective on weight loss

Traditional Chinese Medicine (TCM) takes a holistic approach to weight loss, considering not only what we eat, but also the underlying emotional and energetic factors that may contribute to weight gain. Here are some TCM perspectives on weight loss:

The concept of Qi

In TCM, weight gain is often attributed to an imbalance of Qi, the vital energy that flows throughout the body. Qi can become stagnant or blocked, leading to a sluggish metabolism, digestive issues, and weight gain. TCM practitioners aim to restore the flow of Qi through various techniques, including acupuncture, herbal remedies, and dietary changes.

Emotions and stress

TCM also recognizes the role of emotions and stress in weight gain. Emotional stress can lead to overeating, as well as disruptions in digestion and metabolism. TCM practitioners may recommend stress-reducing techniques like meditation or qigong, as well as herbal remedies like ginseng and licorice root to support the adrenal glands.

Eating for balance

TCM emphasizes the importance of eating for balance and harmony within the body. This means consuming a variety of nutrient-dense foods that are appropriate for your body constitution and level of activity. It also means avoiding foods that are overly processed or difficult to digest, as well as foods that may exacerbate certain health conditions.

The Five Elements

The Five Elements are a key concept in TCM, representing different energetic qualities that are present in nature and the body. Each element corresponds to certain organs and bodily functions, and imbalances in these elements can contribute to weight gain. For example, an excess of Earth element energy may lead to digestive issues and weight gain, while an imbalance in Water element energy may lead to fluid retention and bloating.

Acupuncture

Acupuncture is a popular TCM modality that can be helpful for weight loss. By targeting specific acupressure points on the body, acupuncture can help regulate appetite, boost metabolism, and support healthy digestion and elimination. Some studies have also suggested that acupuncture may help reduce stress and anxiety, which can contribute to weight gain.

Herbal remedies

Herbal remedies are another important aspect of TCM weight loss strategies. Some herbs, like green tea and ginseng, have been shown to boost metabolism and support weight loss. Other herbs, like licorice root and dandelion, can support digestion and elimination, while also reducing inflammation and stress.

TCM dietary strategies for weight management

Traditional Chinese Medicine (TCM) offers various dietary strategies for weight management that can be helpful for individuals seeking a holistic approach to weight loss. Here are some TCM dietary strategies for weight management:

Eating for your body constitution

In TCM, each person has a unique body constitution that determines how they process and metabolize food. By understanding your body constitution, you can make dietary choices that are optimal for your individual needs. For example, those with a Spleen and Stomach deficiency may benefit from warming foods like ginger and cinnamon, while those with a Liver and Gallbladder imbalance may benefit from bitter and sour foods like grapefruit and vinegar.

Eating according to the seasons

TCM also recommends eating according to the seasons to support overall health and balance. During the summer, for example, TCM suggests eating cooling and hydrating foods like watermelon and cucumber, while in the winter, warming foods like root vegetables and soups are recommended. By eating seasonally, we can support our body's natural rhythms and promote balance.

Eating for energy

TCM recognizes that food not only provides nutrition but also energy. Foods are classified according to their energetic properties, such as hot, cold, warm, or cool. By choosing foods that balance and harmonize our energy, we can support overall health and vitality. For example, someone who is always cold and sluggish may benefit from warming foods like ginger and garlic, while someone who is always overheated may benefit from cooling foods like cucumber and watermelon.

Mindful eating

TCM emphasizes the importance of mindful eating, which means paying attention to the texture, taste, and aroma of our food, as well as our hunger and fullness signals. Mindful eating can help us avoid overeating, promote healthy digestion, and support overall wellness. TCM also recommends chewing food thoroughly and eating slowly to aid in digestion and absorption.

Food combinations

TCM also recognizes that certain food combinations can promote healthy digestion and metabolism. For example, combining protein and vegetables can support digestion, while combining protein and starches can slow digestion and lead to bloating. TCM recommends avoiding processed and refined foods and instead choosing whole foods that are minimally processed and easy to digest.

Herbal remedies

Herbal remedies are a key aspect of TCM dietary strategies for weight management. Certain herbs like green tea, ginseng, and licorice root have been shown to support weight loss by boosting metabolism and regulating appetite. Other herbs like ginger, cinnamon, and fennel can support digestion and reduce inflammation, which can contribute to weight gain.

Chapter Twelve

TCM Nutrition for Emotional Well-Being

In Traditional Chinese Medicine (TCM), food is not just seen as a source of nutrition but also as a way to support emotional well-being. TCM practitioners believe that food can impact our emotions and that certain foods can help to balance our emotions and improve overall mental health. Here are some TCM nutrition tips for emotional well-being:

Balance your emotions with food

TCM views emotions as interconnected with physical health, and as such, diet is considered an important factor in regulating emotional balance. Each emotion corresponds to a particular organ and element in TCM theory, and specific foods can be chosen to regulate those emotions. For example, someone with excessive anger or frustration may benefit from cooling foods like cucumber and watermelon, while someone with excessive worry or overthinking may benefit from grounding foods like sweet potato and brown rice.

Choose foods that support relaxation

Certain foods have a calming effect on the mind and body and can be helpful for managing stress and anxiety. TCM recommends incorporating foods that contain tryptophan, an amino acid that supports the production of serotonin, a neurotransmitter that helps regulate mood. Foods that contain tryptophan include turkey, chicken, fish, tofu, pumpkin seeds, and bananas. Other foods that have a calming effect include chamomile tea, lavender, and valerian root.

Eat a balanced diet

A balanced diet that includes a variety of nutrient-dense foods is essential for overall emotional well-being. In TCM, it is recommended to eat a diet that is 70% plant-based and includes a variety of whole foods like fruits, vegetables, whole grains, and lean protein sources. Eating a balanced diet can help to regulate blood sugar levels and support healthy brain function, which can improve emotional stability.

Avoid processed and refined foods

Processed and refined foods are often high in sugar, salt, and unhealthy fats, which can negatively impact emotional well-being. These foods can cause spikes in blood sugar levels and lead to energy crashes, mood swings, and irritability. In TCM, it is recommended to avoid processed and refined foods and instead choose whole foods that are minimally processed and easy to digest.

Mindful eating

Practicing mindful eating can also be helpful for emotional well-being. By paying attention to our hunger and fullness signals and practicing mindful eating, we can improve our relationship with food and reduce emotional eating. TCM also recommends taking the time to prepare and cook meals mindfully, as this can be a form of meditation and stress relief.

Herbal remedies

Herbal remedies are a key aspect of TCM nutrition for emotional well-being. Certain herbs like chamomile, ashwagandha, and lemon balm have calming and stress-reducing properties, while others like ginseng and licorice root can support energy and vitality. TCM practitioners may recommend herbal remedies to help balance emotions and support overall mental health.

The connection between diet and emotions

The concept of food and emotions is not new, as many people often turn to food for comfort or to lift their mood. However, Traditional Chinese Medicine (TCM) takes this connection to another level, viewing food as a critical component of emotional well-being. According to TCM, emotions can significantly impact physical health and vice versa, and food can play a vital role in balancing emotions and promoting overall well-being.

TCM believes that emotions and physical health are interconnected, and imbalances in either can lead to health problems. Each emotion is associated with a particular organ, and excessive or prolonged emotions can damage that organ. For example, the liver is associated with anger, the heart with joy, the spleen with worry, the lungs with grief, and the kidneys with fear. Therefore, if one experiences prolonged or excessive anger, it can affect the liver's function, leading to liver-related health problems.

TCM also acknowledges that certain foods have specific energetic properties that can affect emotions. For example, foods that are too cold or too hot can impact emotions negatively. Similarly, an imbalance in taste preferences can cause imbalances in emotions. For example, excessive consumption of bitter foods can cause feelings of irritability, while too much sweetness can lead to sluggishness and lack of motivation.

To balance emotions and promote overall well-being, TCM emphasizes eating a diet that includes a variety of whole, fresh, seasonal, and locally grown foods. TCM also recommends choosing foods with appropriate tastes and temperatures that support one's body's needs and constitution.

Here are some TCM dietary recommendations to promote emotional well-being:

1. Eat a Balanced Diet: TCM recommends consuming a balanced diet that includes all the essential nutrients in the right proportions. A balanced diet should include whole grains, fresh fruits and vegetables, lean protein, and healthy fats. Avoid processed and refined foods that can cause imbalances in emotions.

2. Consume Warm Foods: Warm foods, such as soups, stews, and warm teas, can help promote feelings of warmth and comfort. These foods can be particularly beneficial during the colder months when many people experience feelings of sadness or depression.

3. Choose the Right Tastes: TCM recommends balancing all five tastes in one's diet: sweet, sour, bitter, salty, and pungent. Each taste has unique properties that can affect emotions. For example, sweet foods can promote a sense of calm and grounding, while sour foods can help to relieve frustration.

4. Incorporate Specific Foods: Certain foods have properties that can benefit specific emotions. For example, green leafy vegetables can help to reduce stress and promote feelings of relaxation. Nuts and seeds are rich in healthy fats that can help to boost mood and brain function. Turmeric and ginger have anti-inflammatory properties that can help to reduce anxiety and promote calmness.

5. Consider Herbal Remedies: TCM uses herbal remedies to promote emotional well-being. Herbs such as St. John's Wort, ashwagandha, and passionflower have properties that can help to reduce anxiety and stress.

Foods that support emotional balance

Traditional Chinese Medicine (TCM) emphasizes the connection between the mind and body, and considers the emotional state to be an essential aspect of overall health. TCM nutrition recognizes that what we eat can have a profound impact on our emotions and moods. Certain foods are believed to have the ability to calm the mind, lift the spirits, and promote emotional balance.

In TCM, each food has its own unique properties and energetics, which can be classified into categories of hot, warm, neutral, cool, and cold. Some foods are believed to have a direct impact on the emotions, while others support the organs that are related to emotional balance.

Here are some foods that are recommended for emotional balance in TCM nutrition:

1. Bitter Foods: Bitter foods are believed to have a cooling effect on the body and are associated with the Heart and Small Intestine meridians in TCM. Foods such as bitter melon, dandelion greens, and arugula are believed to help calm the mind and relieve stress.

2. Sour Foods: Sour foods are believed to have an astringent effect on the body and are associated with the Liver and Gallbladder meridians in TCM. Foods such as lemons, vinegar, and pickles are believed to help relieve irritability and promote a sense of calm.

3. Sweet Foods: Sweet foods are believed to have a tonifying effect on the body and are associated with the Spleen and Stomach meridians in TCM. Foods such as sweet potatoes, carrots, and winter squash are believed to help nourish the body and promote emotional stability.

4. Salty Foods: Salty foods are believed to have a moistening effect on the body and are associated with the Kidney and Bladder meridians in TCM.

Foods such as miso, seaweed, and soy sauce are believed to help calm the mind and promote a sense of grounding.

5. Warm Foods: Warm foods are believed to have a stimulating effect on the body and are associated with the Spleen and Stomach meridians in TCM. Foods such as ginger, cinnamon, and garlic are believed to help warm the body and promote a sense of comfort.

6. Cooling Foods: Cooling foods are believed to have a calming effect on the body and are associated with the Liver and Gallbladder meridians in TCM. Foods such as watermelon, cucumber, and mint are believed to help cool the body and promote a sense of relaxation.

In addition to incorporating these specific foods into the diet, TCM nutrition also emphasizes the importance of eating a balanced diet that includes a variety of whole foods. Eating regular meals, avoiding processed foods and refined sugars, and staying hydrated are also important for emotional balance.

Furthermore, TCM nutrition recommends avoiding excess intake of caffeine, alcohol, and spicy foods, as they can overstimulate the body and lead to feelings of anxiety and restlessness. Eating a variety of colors in meals is also important to ensure a range of nutrients and to support overall health.

Chapter Thirteen

TCM Nutrition for Energy and Vitality

TCM (Traditional Chinese Medicine) Nutrition is a holistic approach to health and wellness that emphasizes the importance of using food as medicine. In TCM, food is seen not only as a source of nourishment but also as a means of promoting balance and harmony within the body. By consuming the right foods in the right amounts and combinations, we can support our body's natural energy and vitality, allowing us to feel our best both physically and mentally.

One of the key principles of TCM Nutrition is the concept of Qi, which refers to the life force or energy that flows through all living things. In TCM, it is believed that the food we eat can either support or deplete our Qi, depending on its quality and properties. Foods that are fresh, whole, and nutrient-dense are considered to be high in Qi and are thought to support the body's natural energy and vitality. On the other hand, foods that are processed, refined, or high in sugar and unhealthy fats are believed to be low in Qi and can deplete our energy over time.

Another important principle of TCM Nutrition is the concept of Yin and Yang. These are opposing forces that exist in all things, including food. Yin is associated with coolness, moisture, and inwardness, while Yang is associated with warmth, dryness, and outwardness. In order to maintain balance and harmony in the body, it is important to consume foods that have a balance of Yin and Yang energies.

In TCM Nutrition, there are also specific foods that are believed to support energy and vitality. These include:

1. Whole grains: Whole grains are considered to be an excellent source of complex carbohydrates, which provide the body with sustained energy throughout the day. Examples of whole grains include brown rice, quinoa, and oats.

2. Leafy greens: Leafy greens, such as spinach, kale, and collard greens, are rich in vitamins and minerals that support overall health and energy.

3. Root vegetables: Root vegetables, such as sweet potatoes, carrots, and beets, are believed to support the body's Qi and promote overall energy and vitality.

4. Nuts and seeds: Nuts and seeds are a great source of healthy fats, protein, and fiber, which can help to support energy levels and keep us feeling full and satisfied.

5. Lean proteins: Lean proteins, such as chicken, fish, and tofu, are an important part of a balanced diet and can provide the body with the amino acids it needs to maintain muscle mass and support energy levels.

In addition to these foods, there are also specific TCM herbs that are believed to support energy and vitality. These include:

6. Ginseng: Ginseng is a popular TCM herb that is believed to support energy levels and improve mental clarity and focus.

7. Astragalus: Astragalus is a root herb that is believed to support overall health and vitality, as well as boost the immune system.

8. Schisandra: Schisandra is a berry that is believed to have adaptogenic properties, meaning it can help the body adapt to stress and support overall energy and vitality.

When it comes to TCM Nutrition for energy and vitality, it is important to focus on consuming a balanced diet that includes a variety of whole, nutrient-dense foods. In addition, incorporating TCM herbs and supplements can also be a helpful way to support energy levels and overall health. By taking a holistic approach to nutrition and considering the energetic properties of food, we can support our body's natural energy and vitality and feel our best both physically and mentally.

Foods that boost Qi

Traditional Chinese Medicine (TCM) emphasizes the importance of Qi, which can be described as the vital energy that flows throughout the body. It is believed that when Qi is in balance and flowing smoothly, we experience good health and vitality. However, when Qi becomes blocked or deficient, we may experience a variety of health problems, such as fatigue, weakness, and decreased immunity. TCM nutrition can play a role in supporting and boosting Qi levels by incorporating foods that are believed to have Qi-boosting properties.

One of the most commonly recommended foods for boosting Qi in TCM is ginseng. Ginseng is believed to be an adaptogen, which means it helps the body adapt to stress and improves overall vitality. It is often recommended for individuals who are fatigued or experiencing low energy levels. Ginseng can be consumed in a variety of forms, including tea, capsules, or as an ingredient in soups and stews.

Another popular Qi-boosting food in TCM is astragalus root. Astragalus is believed to be a powerful immune system booster and is often used to support overall vitality and stamina. It can be consumed as a tea or as an ingredient in soups and stews.

Mushrooms are also considered to be a Qi-boosting food in TCM, particularly varieties such as shiitake and reishi. These mushrooms contain beta-glucans, which are believed to have immune-boosting properties. Additionally, they are believed to have adaptogenic properties and can help improve overall vitality and energy levels.

TCM also places a strong emphasis on the importance of nourishing the blood as a means of supporting Qi levels. Foods that are rich in iron and other nutrients that support blood production, such as leafy green vegetables and red meat, are often recommended for individuals experiencing Qi deficiencies.

In addition to specific foods, TCM also recommends certain dietary habits and practices to support Qi levels. It is recommended to eat slowly and mindfully, chewing food thoroughly to aid in digestion and absorption of nutrients. Eating regular, balanced meals throughout the day can also help maintain stable Qi levels and avoid energy crashes.

TCM also emphasizes the importance of avoiding foods that can deplete Qi levels. Foods that are excessively cold or raw, such as salads and raw vegetables, are believed to weaken the digestive system and may lead to Qi deficiencies. Additionally, overly processed or refined foods are believed to be difficult to digest and may contribute to Qi imbalances.

Dietary tips for sustained energy

Diet plays a crucial role in determining our energy levels throughout the day. Traditional Chinese Medicine (TCM) offers dietary tips that can help us sustain our energy levels throughout the day. According to TCM, our diet can affect our Qi (pronounced chee), the vital energy that flows through our body, and is responsible for maintaining our physical and mental well-being. Here are some dietary tips for sustained energy from a TCM perspective.

Eat a balanced diet

1. A balanced diet is essential to maintain optimal energy levels throughout the day. A balanced diet includes foods from all five food groups: grains, vegetables, fruits, proteins, and fats. Each food group has a unique role to play in providing energy to the body. Grains provide carbohydrates, which are the primary source of energy for the body. Vegetables and fruits provide essential vitamins and minerals that are essential for energy production. Proteins help to build and repair muscles, which is crucial for energy production. Fats provide long-lasting energy to the body and also help to absorb fat-soluble vitamins.

Avoid processed foods

Processed foods are high in sugar, salt, and fat and can cause a spike in blood sugar levels, leading to a sudden crash in energy levels. Processed foods are also low in essential nutrients such as vitamins, minerals, and fiber, which are essential for energy production. Instead, opt for whole foods that are nutrient-dense and provide sustained energy throughout the day.

Eat foods that boost Qi

According to TCM, certain foods can boost Qi and provide sustained energy throughout the day. Foods that boost Qi include:

Root vegetables such as sweet potato, carrot, and beetroot

Whole grains such as brown rice, quinoa, and millet

Leafy greens such as kale, spinach, and collard greens

Fruits such as apples, berries, and oranges

Nuts and seeds such as almonds, walnuts, and pumpkin seeds

Legumes such as lentils, chickpeas, and black beans

Eat small, frequent meals

Eating small, frequent meals throughout the day can help to maintain steady blood sugar levels and prevent energy crashes. Eating small, frequent meals also helps to keep the metabolism active and promotes sustained energy production.

Drink plenty of water

Water is essential for maintaining optimal energy levels throughout the day. Dehydration can cause fatigue, headache, and dizziness, which can affect our energy levels. Drinking plenty of water can help to prevent dehydration and maintain optimal energy levels.

Eat warm, cooked foods

According to TCM, eating warm, cooked foods can help to boost Qi and provide sustained energy throughout the day. Raw, cold foods are believed to weaken the digestive system and can lead to a lack of energy. Eating warm, cooked foods, on the other hand, is believed to nourish the digestive system and promote energy production.

Eat mindfully

Eating mindfully can help to improve digestion and promote sustained energy production. Mindful eating involves paying attention to the taste, texture, and aroma of the food and taking the time to chew slowly and thoroughly. Mindful eating also involves avoiding distractions such as TV, mobile phones, and computers while eating.

Chapter Fourteen

TCM Nutrition for Women's Health

Traditional Chinese Medicine (TCM) has been used for centuries to address women's health issues. TCM emphasizes the importance of a balanced diet that considers the body's constitution and the energetic properties of foods. Below we will explore TCM nutrition for women's health, including the common issues that women face, the specific dietary recommendations, and the herbs and supplements that can support women's health.

Women's Health Issues in TCM

TCM recognizes that women's health is influenced by various factors, including the menstrual cycle, childbirth, and menopause. The TCM approach to women's health emphasizes the balance of Yin and Yang, the two opposing forces that regulate the body's functions.

In TCM, women's health issues are often related to the stagnation or deficiency of Qi, blood, or both. Common issues include menstrual cramps, irregular periods, menopause symptoms, and infertility.

Dietary Recommendations for Women's Health

TCM nutrition for women's health focuses on promoting the balance of Yin and Yang and supporting the body's vital substances, such as Qi and blood. Here are some dietary recommendations that can support women's health:

Eat warming foods

In TCM, women are believed to have a colder constitution than men, which makes them more prone to Qi and blood stagnation. Therefore, eating warming foods can help to promote circulation and prevent stagnation. Warming foods include ginger, cinnamon, garlic, and pepper.

Consume blood-nourishing foods

Since blood deficiency is a common issue for women, consuming foods that nourish the blood can be helpful. These foods include dark leafy greens, beets, liver, and red meat.

Eat Qi-tonifying foods

Qi deficiency is another common issue for women, and consuming Qi-tonifying foods can help to support energy levels. These foods include whole grains, beans, nuts, and seeds.

Incorporate Yin-nourishing foods

Yin deficiency can manifest as dryness in the body, including the skin, hair, and mucous membranes. Incorporating Yin-nourishing foods, such as tofu, black beans, and seaweed, can help to moisten and nourish the body.

Herbs and Supplements for Women's Health

In addition to dietary recommendations, TCM also uses herbs and supplements to support women's health. Here are some common herbs and supplements used in TCM:

Dong Quai

Dong Quai, also known as Angelica sinensis, is a herb commonly used in TCM for women's health. It is believed to nourish the blood, regulate the menstrual cycle, and alleviate menstrual cramps.

Shatavari

Shatavari, also known as Asparagus racemosus, is a herb commonly used in Ayurveda and TCM for women's health. It is believed to nourish the Yin, support reproductive health, and alleviate menopause symptoms.

Red Raspberry Leaf

Red Raspberry Leaf is a herb commonly used in Western herbalism and TCM for women's health. It is believed to tone the uterus, promote fertility, and alleviate menstrual cramps.

Iron supplements

Since women are more prone to blood deficiency, iron supplements can be helpful to support healthy blood levels. Iron-rich foods include red meat, liver, and dark leafy greens.

TCM dietary recommendations for menstrual health

TCM or Traditional Chinese Medicine is a holistic approach to healthcare that emphasizes the importance of maintaining balance and harmony within the body. In TCM, diet is seen as an essential component of maintaining health and preventing illness. As such, TCM has specific dietary recommendations for various health conditions, including menstrual health.

Menstruation is a natural process that occurs in women of reproductive age. However, for some women, menstruation can be accompanied by discomfort, pain, and other symptoms that can affect their quality of life. TCM offers a holistic approach to managing menstrual health that involves dietary recommendations, herbal remedies, and lifestyle modifications.

According to TCM, the menstrual cycle is closely linked to the concept of Qi, or vital energy, and blood. Qi and blood are believed to flow through meridians, or pathways, throughout the body, and any disruption in the flow of Qi or blood can lead to menstrual irregularities and other health problems.

To support menstrual health, TCM dietary recommendations focus on nourishing the blood and promoting the flow of Qi. Here are some TCM dietary tips for menstrual health:

1. Eat Warm Foods: In TCM, the menstrual cycle is associated with the element of Water and the Kidney organ. Eating warm and nourishing foods, such as soups, stews, and warm grains, can help support the Kidney and promote the flow of Qi and blood.

2. Consume Iron-rich Foods: Blood is a crucial component of the menstrual cycle, and it is essential to nourish the blood to support a healthy cycle. Iron is an essential nutrient for blood production, and consuming iron-rich foods, such as dark leafy greens, red meat, and beans, can help support blood production.

3. Avoid Cold Foods and Drinks: In TCM, cold foods and drinks are believed to slow down the flow of Qi and blood, leading to menstrual cramps and other symptoms. Therefore, it is recommended to avoid cold foods and drinks during menstruation and opt for warm or room temperature foods instead.

4. Incorporate Blood-tonifying Foods: In TCM, there are specific foods believed to nourish the blood and support menstrual health. These include red dates, goji berries, black sesame seeds, and bone broth.

5. Reduce Processed Foods and Sugar: Processed foods and sugar can disrupt the flow of Qi and blood, leading to menstrual irregularities and other health problems. It is recommended to reduce the intake of processed foods and sugar and opt for whole, nutrient-dense foods instead.

In addition to dietary recommendations, TCM also utilizes herbal remedies to support menstrual health. Herbs such as Dong Quai, Shu Di Huang, and Bai Shao are believed to nourish the blood and regulate menstrual cycles.

TCM nutrition for fertility and pregnancy

TCM (Traditional Chinese Medicine) has a holistic approach to healthcare, where dietary and lifestyle factors are considered important to overall health and wellbeing. This is particularly true when it comes to fertility and pregnancy, where TCM has a wealth of knowledge about how to optimize nutrition to support reproductive health.

In TCM, it is believed that the body has a continuous flow of energy or Qi, which is responsible for regulating the reproductive organs. When Qi is flowing freely, the reproductive system functions optimally, and fertility is enhanced. TCM nutrition seeks to optimize Qi by balancing the Yin and Yang energies, which help to regulate hormones and the menstrual cycle.

One of the key dietary recommendations for fertility is to ensure adequate blood and nutrient supply to the reproductive organs. Blood is considered a Yin substance in TCM, and is responsible for nourishing the organs and tissues. Foods that are rich in iron, folate, and other B-vitamins, such as dark leafy greens, lentils, and liver, can help to build blood and support fertility.

Another important aspect of TCM nutrition for fertility is to support the Kidney Qi. The Kidney is considered the foundation of the reproductive system, and supporting its Qi is essential for optimal fertility. Foods that are rich in Zinc, such as oysters, nuts, and seeds, are important for Kidney Qi, as are foods that are rich in essential fatty acids, such as oily fish, avocado, and flaxseed oil.

During pregnancy, TCM nutrition focuses on supporting the developing fetus, as well as the health of the mother. In TCM, pregnancy is considered a Yin state, where the body's resources are directed towards nourishing and supporting the growth of the baby. As such, it is important to eat foods that are nutrient-dense, and that can help to support the developing fetus.

Foods that are rich in protein, such as eggs, lean meats, and legumes, are important for fetal growth and development. It is also important to eat a variety of colorful fruits and vegetables, which provide essential vitamins and minerals, such as Vitamin C and folate.

In TCM, it is believed that the digestive system is closely linked to the health of the mother and baby during pregnancy. Foods that are easy to digest, such as soups and stews, are often recommended during pregnancy, as they can help to support digestive function and promote nutrient absorption. It is also important to avoid foods that are too spicy or greasy, as they can cause digestive upset.

In addition to dietary recommendations, TCM also emphasizes the importance of a balanced lifestyle during pregnancy. This includes getting adequate rest, avoiding stress, and engaging in gentle exercise, such as yoga or walking.

Chapter Fifteen

TCM Nutrition for Men's Health

Traditional Chinese Medicine (TCM) emphasizes the importance of maintaining balance and harmony within the body to achieve optimal health. TCM nutrition plays a vital role in achieving this balance and is based on the individual's constitution, their stage in life, and any underlying health concerns they may have. While TCM nutrition may differ from Western nutrition, both focus on nourishing the body with nutrient-dense foods.

When it comes to men's health, TCM focuses on maintaining the balance of the body's vital energy, or Qi. One of the fundamental concepts in TCM is the idea of Yin and Yang, where Yin represents the body's cooling and nourishing properties, while Yang represents the body's warming and energizing properties. A balance of these two energies is crucial for men's health, and TCM nutrition can help achieve this balance.

One of the primary concerns in men's health is maintaining prostate health. TCM nutrition emphasizes the importance of including foods that are beneficial to the prostate, such as pumpkin seeds, tomatoes, and soy products. These foods contain lycopene, an antioxidant that has been shown to reduce the risk of prostate cancer. Additionally, TCM suggests avoiding spicy and greasy foods that can aggravate the prostate and cause inflammation.

TCM also places significant emphasis on the importance of kidney health, as the kidneys are considered the foundation of Qi in the body. TCM recommends including kidney-nourishing foods such as black beans, kidney beans, walnuts, and sesame seeds. These foods are high in essential nutrients such as zinc, which is crucial for the production of testosterone and the maintenance of healthy sperm.

Another essential aspect of men's health is maintaining healthy blood circulation. TCM suggests including foods that promote blood circulation, such as ginger, garlic, and onions. These foods contain compounds that have been shown to improve blood flow and lower blood pressure, reducing the risk of heart disease.

In addition to dietary recommendations, TCM also recommends incorporating lifestyle changes such as regular exercise, stress management techniques, and adequate sleep to promote men's health. These practices help maintain the balance of Qi in the body, reducing the risk of chronic diseases and promoting overall well-being.

TCM dietary recommendations for male vitality

Traditional Chinese Medicine (TCM) offers a holistic approach to health and wellness, including dietary recommendations that are tailored to support specific health concerns. For men's health, TCM emphasizes the importance of maintaining vitality and supporting the body's natural functions. Diet plays a significant role in achieving these goals, and there are several TCM dietary recommendations that can help promote male vitality.

One of the key concepts in TCM is the idea of Qi, or life force energy. In TCM, Qi is believed to flow through the body and support overall health and vitality. To support Qi and maintain vitality, TCM recommends consuming foods that are warm and nourishing, such as whole grains, lean proteins, and cooked vegetables. These foods provide the body with sustained energy and can help support the immune system.

Another important aspect of TCM dietary recommendations for male vitality is the consumption of foods that support the kidneys. In TCM, the kidneys are seen as a vital organ that supports overall health and vitality, including sexual function. Foods that support the kidneys include black beans, kidney beans, walnuts, and seeds like pumpkin and sunflower. These foods are believed to nourish the kidneys and support healthy functioning.

TCM also emphasizes the importance of consuming foods that are rich in nutrients that support male health. For example, foods that are high in zinc, such as oysters, beef, and pumpkin seeds, can help support healthy testosterone levels and promote overall male vitality. Similarly, foods that are high in B vitamins, such as whole grains and leafy greens, can help support energy levels and promote healthy nervous system function.

In addition to specific foods, TCM also recommends certain cooking methods to promote male vitality. For example, TCM recommends using slow-cooking methods like stews and soups to help release the nourishing properties of foods and make them easier to digest. TCM also recommends consuming warm foods and avoiding raw or cold foods, which can be harder for the body to digest and may deplete Qi.

Finally, TCM emphasizes the importance of moderation in all things, including diet. While certain foods and dietary recommendations can support male vitality, excessive consumption of certain foods or overeating can have a negative impact on overall health. TCM recommends eating regular, balanced meals and listening to the body's natural hunger and fullness cues to support overall health and vitality.

TCM nutrition for prostate health

Traditional Chinese Medicine (TCM) has a holistic approach to health, which includes dietary recommendations for specific health concerns. One common health issue that affects many men is prostate health. TCM offers dietary strategies to support prostate health and prevent prostate-related problems.

According to TCM, the prostate is an organ associated with the Kidney and Bladder meridians. These organs are essential in maintaining male reproductive health. The Kidney meridian is responsible for storing Jing, the essence of life, while the Bladder meridian regulates the flow of Qi and fluids in the lower part of the body. In TCM theory, an imbalance in these meridians can lead to prostate problems.

To maintain prostate health, TCM recommends consuming foods that nourish and strengthen the Kidney and Bladder meridians. Here are some dietary tips for prostate health:

1. Eat warming and tonifying foods: In TCM, the Kidney meridian is associated with the element of Water, which is yin in nature. To balance the yin, it is important to consume warming and tonifying foods that are yang in nature. Examples of warming and tonifying foods include lamb, beef, chicken, shrimp, walnuts, chestnuts, ginger, and cinnamon. These foods help to nourish the Kidney meridian and promote circulation of Qi and blood to the prostate.

2. Increase intake of fruits and vegetables: Fruits and vegetables are important sources of antioxidants, vitamins, and minerals that support prostate health. Examples of fruits and vegetables that are beneficial for the prostate include tomatoes, watermelon, pumpkin, carrots, kale, and broccoli. These foods are rich in lycopene, beta-carotene, and vitamin C, which help to reduce inflammation and oxidative stress in the prostate.

3. Avoid spicy and greasy foods: Spicy and greasy foods can exacerbate inflammation and heat in the body, leading to prostate problems. TCM recommends avoiding or reducing the intake of these foods to maintain prostate health.

4. Drink herbal teas: TCM herbs can be brewed into teas to support prostate health. Examples of herbs that are beneficial for the prostate include saw palmetto, nettle root, pygeum, and green tea. These herbs have anti-inflammatory and antioxidant properties that help to reduce the risk of prostate problems.

5. Practice moderation: In TCM, moderation is key to maintaining good health. Overeating, drinking excessive amounts of alcohol, or consuming too much spicy or greasy food can create an imbalance in the body and lead to prostate problems. Eating a balanced diet, practicing portion control, and avoiding overindulgence can help to maintain prostate health.

In addition to these dietary tips, TCM also recommends regular exercise, stress management, and acupuncture to support prostate health. Incorporating these lifestyle practices into your routine can help to maintain overall health and prevent prostate problems.

Chapter Sixteen

TCM Nutrition for Healthy Aging

TCM, or Traditional Chinese Medicine, has a long history of emphasizing the importance of nutrition for overall health and wellness. In TCM, food is seen not only as a source of sustenance, but also as a means of promoting and maintaining the body's balance and harmony. As we age, our bodies go through many changes, and it becomes increasingly important to pay attention to the foods we eat and how they affect our health. Below we will explore the principles of TCM nutrition for healthy aging, including the role of specific foods and herbs in promoting longevity and vitality.

In TCM, the concept of "Qi" (pronounced "chee") is central to understanding how nutrition affects the body. Qi is often translated as "life force" or "vital energy," and is believed to flow through the body's meridians, or energy pathways. When Qi is flowing smoothly and in balance, the body is healthy and vibrant. However, when Qi becomes blocked or stagnant, the body can experience a variety of health problems. TCM nutrition focuses on maintaining the free flow of Qi throughout the body, which is essential for healthy aging.

One of the key principles of TCM nutrition for healthy aging is to eat a balanced diet that includes a variety of foods. In TCM, foods are classified according to their energetic properties, such as hot, warm, neutral, cool, or cold. The goal is to consume a balance of these different energies to maintain overall balance in the body. For example, foods that are classified as "hot" or "warm" are believed to stimulate circulation and metabolism, while "cool" or "cold" foods are thought to have a calming and soothing effect on the body. It is important to note that these classifications are not based on the physical temperature of the food, but rather on their energetic properties.

In addition to balancing the energetic properties of food, TCM nutrition also emphasizes the importance of consuming foods that are rich in nutrients and antioxidants. These include fresh fruits and vegetables, whole grains, lean proteins, and healthy fats. Many of these foods are also high in anti-inflammatory compounds, which can help to protect the body against chronic diseases such as heart disease and cancer.

Certain herbs and supplements are also commonly used in TCM to promote healthy aging. For example, ginseng is a popular herb that is believed to enhance vitality and improve cognitive function. Other herbs, such as goji berries and astragalus, are used for their antioxidant properties and ability to boost the immune system. It is important to note that herbs and supplements should always be used under the guidance of a qualified practitioner, as they can interact with medications and may not be appropriate for everyone.

In addition to following a balanced diet and incorporating herbs and supplements as appropriate, there are several other dietary recommendations that can support healthy aging in TCM. These include:

1. Eating smaller, more frequent meals: In TCM, it is believed that overeating and consuming large meals can put a strain on the digestive system, which can lead to a variety of health problems. Eating smaller, more frequent meals can help to support digestion and prevent digestive issues such as bloating and constipation.

2. Avoiding processed and refined foods: Processed and refined foods are often high in unhealthy fats, sugar, and additives, and are believed to contribute to inflammation and other chronic health conditions. Instead, focus on whole foods that are minimally processed and free from additives.

3. Drinking plenty of water: Adequate hydration is essential for healthy aging, as it helps to support healthy digestion, circulation, and elimination. Aim to drink at least 8 glasses of water per day, and avoid sugary drinks and excessive amounts of caffeine and alcohol.

4. Eating mindfully: Mindful eating is an

TCM dietary recommendations for longevity

Traditional Chinese Medicine (TCM) has been promoting longevity and overall health for thousands of years. In TCM, food is not just a source of nourishment, but also a form of medicine. Therefore, choosing the right foods and eating habits can have a significant impact on one's health and longevity. Below we will explore TCM dietary recommendations for longevity and how to implement them in our daily lives.

TCM views aging as a natural process that is influenced by both internal and external factors. These factors include genetics, lifestyle, environment, and nutrition. In TCM, the concept of "Qi" is often used to describe the body's energy flow, and a healthy diet is crucial for maintaining a balanced Qi. When the Qi is in balance, the body can resist disease, promote healing, and promote longevity.

1. One of the fundamental principles of TCM dietary recommendations for longevity is moderation. TCM suggests that we should not overindulge in any particular food or drink, as excess can cause imbalances in the body. Moreover, a balanced diet should include a variety of foods from all five

taste categories: sweet, sour, salty, bitter, and umami. Each taste has unique properties and can have specific effects on the body.

In TCM, foods that are considered "tonic" are believed to strengthen the body, boost the immune system, and promote longevity. These foods include ginseng, goji berries, astragalus, and shiitake mushrooms. These foods are rich in vitamins, minerals, and antioxidants that help protect the body from damage caused by free radicals.

Another essential aspect of TCM dietary recommendations for longevity is the consumption of foods that support the body's natural detoxification process. Foods such as broccoli, cabbage, kale, and other cruciferous vegetables contain compounds that can help eliminate toxins from the body. Additionally, TCM recommends the consumption of probiotic-rich foods such as sauerkraut, kefir, and yogurt to support the body's natural microbiome.

TCM also emphasizes the importance of maintaining a healthy digestive system. Digestion is a complex process that involves the breakdown of food into nutrients that can be absorbed and used by the body. TCM recommends consuming foods that are easy to digest, such as soups, stews, and congee, to support digestive health. Additionally, TCM suggests avoiding processed and greasy foods that can be difficult for the body to digest.

In TCM, the concept of "yin and yang" is often used to describe the balance of opposing forces in the body. The yin represents the cooling, calming, and nourishing aspects of the body, while the yang represents the warming, stimulating, and energizing aspects. To promote longevity, TCM suggests balancing the yin and yang in the body by consuming foods that are appropriate for one's body type and the current season.

TCM dietary recommendations for longevity also include incorporating herbs into one's diet. Herbs such as ginger, turmeric, and cinnamon are believed to have anti-inflammatory and antioxidant properties that can help protect the body from damage caused by aging. Additionally, TCM recommends consuming herbal teas such as green tea, chrysanthemum tea, and dandelion tea, which are believed to support the body's natural detoxification process and promote longevity.

Foods that nourish the Kidneys and support aging gracefully

Traditional Chinese Medicine (TCM) emphasizes the importance of nourishing the kidneys to support healthy aging. According to TCM principles, the kidneys are the foundation of our vital essence, or "jing," and play a key role in our overall health and longevity. As we age, our kidney energy naturally declines, making it essential to nourish and support this vital organ through diet and lifestyle choices. Below we will explore some of the best foods to nourish the kidneys and support graceful aging.

One of the best ways to nourish the kidneys is by consuming foods that are high in "jing" or essence. In TCM, foods that are rich in jing are believed to help replenish our kidney energy, support healthy aging, and promote longevity. Examples of foods that are high in jing include:

1. Seafood: Seafood is a rich source of protein, omega-3 fatty acids, and minerals such as zinc and selenium, all of which are beneficial for the kidneys. Fish such as salmon, sardines, and mackerel are particularly high in omega-3s and are believed to nourish the kidneys and promote healthy aging.

2. Bone Broth: Bone broth is a nutrient-dense liquid that is made by simmering bones and connective tissue for several hours. This process extracts the nutrients and minerals from the bones, including calcium, magnesium, and phosphorus, which are essential for bone health and kidney function.

Bone broth is also high in collagen, a protein that supports joint health and skin elasticity.

3. Black Beans: Black beans are a staple of traditional Chinese cuisine and are considered one of the best foods for nourishing the kidneys. They are rich in antioxidants, fiber, and protein, and are a good source of minerals such as iron, magnesium, and potassium. Black beans are also believed to help regulate blood sugar levels and support cardiovascular health.

4. Nuts and Seeds: Nuts and seeds are a rich source of healthy fats, protein, and minerals such as zinc and magnesium. Almonds, walnuts, and pumpkin seeds are particularly beneficial for the kidneys and are believed to help support healthy aging and promote longevity.

5. Goji Berries: Goji berries are a small, red berry that are commonly used in TCM to nourish the kidneys and support overall health. They are rich in antioxidants, vitamins, and minerals, and are believed to help support healthy immune function and improve cognitive function.

In addition to these specific foods, there are also certain dietary principles that can help to support kidney health and promote healthy aging. For example, TCM recommends that individuals limit their intake of cold and raw foods, as these can weaken the digestive system and impair kidney function. Instead, it is recommended to consume warm, cooked foods that are easy to digest and nourishing to the kidneys.

TCM also recommends avoiding excessive consumption of foods that are overly sweet, salty, or spicy, as these can contribute to imbalances in the body and weaken kidney energy. Instead, it is recommended to consume a balanced diet that includes a variety of whole foods, including fruits, vegetables, whole grains, and lean proteins.

Finally, TCM emphasizes the importance of mindful eating and the connection between food and emotional well-being. In TCM, it is believed that emotions such as stress, anxiety, and anger can have a negative impact on the kidneys and contribute to imbalances in the body. To support healthy aging, it is recommended to eat in a calm and relaxed state, and to cultivate a positive and peaceful mindset towards food and nutrition.

Chapter Seventeen

TCM Nutrition for Children and Adolescents

TCM (Traditional Chinese Medicine) has been used for thousands of years to promote health and well-being in people of all ages. When it comes to children and adolescents, TCM nutrition can play an important role in supporting growth and development, improving immune function, and preventing or managing health conditions.

In TCM, children and adolescents are considered to have a delicate constitution and their nutritional needs are believed to be different from those of adults. As such, TCM practitioners often tailor their dietary recommendations to the specific needs of younger individuals.

One of the key principles of TCM nutrition for children and adolescents is to promote a balanced diet that includes a variety of foods. TCM considers each food to have specific energetic properties, such as hot, cold, warm, or cool, which can impact the body in different ways. A balanced diet should include foods with a range of energetic properties to maintain overall health and prevent imbalances.

In addition to promoting a balanced diet, TCM nutrition for children and adolescents often includes specific foods and herbs that can support growth and development. For example, foods that are rich in calcium and vitamin D, such as dairy products, leafy greens, and fish, can support strong bones and teeth.

TCM also recognizes the importance of the digestive system in maintaining overall health, and recommends foods that are easy to digest and promote healthy digestion. Foods that are easy to digest, such as soups and stews, are often recommended for children and adolescents who may have weaker digestive systems.

Another important aspect of TCM nutrition for children and adolescents is the concept of seasonal eating. TCM believes that different seasons require different types of foods to support the body's needs. For example, in the winter months, warming foods such as soups and stews are recommended to help the body stay warm and nourished.

TCM nutrition can also play a role in preventing and managing health conditions in children and adolescents. For example, TCM recognizes that many children and adolescents may have weaker immune systems and may be more susceptible to colds and other illnesses. Certain foods and herbs, such as ginger and astragalus, are believed to have immune-boosting properties and can be recommended to support immune function.

Additionally, TCM recognizes that children and adolescents may experience emotional and behavioral imbalances, such as anxiety and hyperactivity. Certain foods and herbs, such as chamomile and oats, are believed to have calming properties and can be recommended to support emotional and behavioral health.

TCM dietary recommendations for growth and development

Traditional Chinese Medicine (TCM) offers a holistic approach to health and wellness, which includes dietary recommendations to support growth and development in children and adolescents. TCM recognizes that children have unique nutritional needs to support their physical, mental, and emotional development. These dietary recommendations focus on maintaining a balance between Yin and Yang energies in the body and supporting the child's vital energy or Qi.

In TCM, the Spleen and Stomach are considered the foundation of a healthy digestive system, which is essential for growth and development. Children are believed to have a weaker digestive system than adults, and their ability to absorb nutrients is not fully developed. Therefore, it is important to provide nutrient-dense foods that are easy to digest.

One of the primary dietary recommendations for children and adolescents is to consume a variety of nutrient-dense foods. TCM practitioners often recommend including foods from all five taste categories (sweet, sour, salty, bitter, and pungent) in a child's diet to ensure a balance of Yin and Yang energies. For example, sweet foods, such as grains, root vegetables, and fruits, are believed to nourish the body and promote digestion. Sour foods, such as vinegar and fermented foods, can stimulate digestion and help balance the Qi. Salty foods, such as seaweed and miso, can help promote the absorption of nutrients, while bitter foods, such as leafy greens, can help cleanse and detoxify the body. Pungent foods, such as ginger and garlic, can help warm and invigorate the body.

Another key recommendation is to focus on whole foods and avoid processed and refined foods. Whole foods, such as fruits, vegetables, whole grains, and lean proteins, provide a wide range of nutrients, including vitamins, minerals, and fiber, which are essential for growth and development. Processed and refined foods, on the other hand, are often high in sugar, salt, and unhealthy fats, which can disrupt the balance of Yin and Yang energies in the body.

TCM also recommends consuming warm, cooked foods over cold and raw foods. Warm, cooked foods are easier to digest and promote healthy Qi flow in the body. In contrast, cold and raw foods can weaken the digestive system and disrupt the balance of Yin and Yang energies. Therefore, it is important to cook food thoroughly and avoid consuming excessive amounts of raw fruits and vegetables.

In addition to dietary recommendations, TCM also emphasizes the importance of eating in a relaxed and peaceful environment. Eating in a calm and relaxed setting can promote healthy digestion and help balance the Qi. Children should be encouraged to eat at regular intervals and avoid eating when stressed, upset, or distracted.

Finally, TCM recognizes the importance of balancing physical activity with rest and relaxation. Children and adolescents should be encouraged to engage in moderate physical activity regularly, such as playing outside, participating in sports, or practicing martial arts. However, it is also essential to allow for adequate rest and relaxation, as this can help balance the Qi and support growth and development.

Foods that support focus and cognitive function

The food we eat has a significant impact on our mental performance, including our ability to focus and think clearly. In Traditional Chinese Medicine (TCM), certain foods are believed to have a direct effect on cognitive function and can help support mental clarity and focus. Below we will explore some of the foods that are believed to be beneficial for cognitive function and the TCM principles behind them.

In TCM, the mind and body are not considered separate entities, but rather part of an interconnected whole. The spleen and stomach play a crucial role in the proper functioning of the brain and the production of Qi (vital energy) and blood. Therefore, it is essential to ensure that these organs are functioning optimally by consuming foods that are easy to digest, nutrient-dense, and nourishing.

One food that is believed to support cognitive function in TCM is walnuts. In TCM, walnuts are considered a brain food due to their high content of omega-3 fatty acids, which are essential for brain health. Walnuts are also rich in vitamin E, which has been shown to have a positive impact on cognitive function. Additionally, walnuts are believed to nourish the kidneys, which are associated with cognitive function in TCM.

Another food that is believed to support cognitive function is blueberries. Blueberries are rich in antioxidants, which help to protect the brain from oxidative stress and inflammation. In TCM, blueberries are considered to be cooling and nourishing, making them an excellent food for promoting mental clarity and focus.

Leafy greens are another food that is believed to be beneficial for cognitive function. In TCM, leafy greens are considered to be cooling and moistening, which makes them an excellent food for promoting mental clarity and focus. Additionally, leafy greens are rich in vitamins and minerals, including folate, which is essential for brain health.

In TCM, it is also believed that consuming warm, cooked foods is better for cognitive function than consuming raw, cold foods. This is because warm, cooked foods are easier to digest and allow the body to more efficiently extract nutrients. Conversely, consuming cold, raw foods can weaken the digestive system and impair the body's ability to absorb nutrients, which can negatively impact cognitive function.

Furthermore, TCM principles suggest that overconsumption of sweet, greasy, and processed foods can lead to an imbalance in the body, resulting in sluggishness and poor cognitive function. Instead, it is recommended to consume a balanced diet that includes a variety of whole foods, including fruits, vegetables, whole grains, and lean proteins.

Chapter Eighteen

Cooking Techniques in TCM Nutrition

Cooking techniques play an essential role in Traditional Chinese Medicine (TCM) nutrition. In TCM, the way food is cooked can impact its energetic properties and how it affects the body. By using certain cooking techniques, we can increase or decrease the energy of a food to balance the body's internal environment. Here, we will explore some of the most common cooking techniques used in TCM nutrition and their benefits.

Steaming

Steaming is one of the most popular cooking techniques in TCM nutrition. Steaming is a gentle cooking method that helps to retain the food's nutritional value, flavor, and color. Steaming is especially beneficial for foods that are considered cooling, such as leafy greens, which help to clear heat and detoxify the body. Steaming is also used for foods that are considered neutral or warming, such as grains and root vegetables.

Boiling

Boiling is another cooking technique that is commonly used in TCM nutrition. Boiling is particularly beneficial for extracting the nutrients and medicinal properties from herbs, roots, and bones. Boiling can help to release the essence of the food, making it easier for the body to digest and absorb its nutrients. In TCM, boiling is often used to make soups and stews, which are known for their nourishing and restorative properties.

Stir-Frying

Stir-frying is a popular cooking technique in Chinese cuisine that is used in TCM nutrition to balance the body's internal environment. Stir-frying involves cooking food over high heat in a small amount of oil for a short period. Stir-frying is particularly beneficial for foods that are considered warming, such as ginger and garlic. Stir-frying can help to increase the energy of a food, making it easier for the body to digest and absorb.

Braising

Braising is a cooking technique that involves cooking food slowly in a small amount of liquid. Braising is used in TCM nutrition to make tough meats and vegetables more tender and easier to digest. Braising is also beneficial for foods that are considered neutral or warming, such as grains and root vegetables. Braising helps to release the essence of the food, making it easier for the body to digest and absorb its nutrients.

Baking

Baking is a cooking technique that is used in TCM nutrition to help increase the energy of a food. Baking involves cooking food in an oven or over an open flame. Baking is particularly beneficial for foods that are considered cooling, such as fruits and vegetables. Baking can help to increase the energy of these foods, making them easier for the body to digest and absorb.

Simmering

Simmering is a cooking technique that involves cooking food over low heat for an extended period. Simmering is often used in TCM nutrition to make broths and soups. Simmering is beneficial for foods that are considered neutral or warming, such as grains and root vegetables. Simmering helps to release the essence of the food, making it easier for the body to digest and absorb its nutrients.

The impact of cooking methods on food properties

The way we prepare our food can have a significant impact on its nutritional properties. In Traditional Chinese Medicine (TCM), cooking techniques are seen as an important aspect of TCM nutrition, with different methods being used to balance the body's internal environment and support overall health.

One key concept in TCM nutrition is the concept of Qi, or vital energy. According to TCM, the way food is cooked can impact its Qi, and therefore its therapeutic effects on the body. For example, TCM suggests that foods cooked at high temperatures for long periods of time can deplete their Qi and reduce their nutritional value.

Another important consideration is the temperature of the cooking method. TCM categorizes foods as hot, warm, neutral, cool, or cold based on their energetic properties. Foods that are hot or warm in nature are thought to be stimulating and can help to warm the body and increase circulation. Cool or cold foods, on the other hand, are thought to be cooling and can help to reduce inflammation and promote relaxation. TCM suggests that cooking methods should be chosen based on the energetic nature of the food being cooked in order to maintain its therapeutic properties.

Steaming is one cooking method that is frequently recommended in TCM nutrition. This method involves cooking food with steam, which can help to preserve its nutritional value and natural flavors. Steaming is particularly beneficial for cooking vegetables, as it can help to soften them without breaking down their cell walls and destroying their nutrients.

Boiling is another cooking method that is commonly used in TCM nutrition. This method involves cooking food in a pot of boiling water, which can help to soften it and make it easier to digest. Boiling is often used for cooking grains, beans, and root vegetables, as it can help to break down their tough fibers and make them more accessible to the body's digestive system.

Stir-frying is a popular cooking method in Chinese cuisine, and is also used in TCM nutrition. This method involves cooking food in a wok or frying pan with a small amount of oil, and can help to preserve the food's natural flavors and textures. Stir-frying is often used for cooking vegetables, as it can help to retain their crispness and natural colors.

Baking is another cooking method that can be used in TCM nutrition, particularly for cooking meats and root vegetables. This method involves cooking food in an oven, and can help to preserve its natural flavors and moisture. However, TCM suggests that baking should be used sparingly, as high temperatures can deplete the food's Qi and reduce its nutritional value.

In addition to these cooking methods, TCM nutrition also emphasizes the importance of using fresh, seasonal ingredients and avoiding processed foods. TCM suggests that foods that are in season are naturally better suited to support the body's needs, and can help to promote balance and harmony within the body.

Choosing the right cooking techniques for balance

Choosing the right cooking techniques for balance is an important aspect of Traditional Chinese Medicine (TCM) nutrition. Cooking methods can greatly affect the energy and nutrient properties of food, and the choice of cooking technique can determine whether a dish is warming, cooling, or neutral. Below we will discuss the various cooking techniques used in TCM nutrition and how to choose the right one for achieving balance.

Steaming is a popular cooking technique in TCM nutrition. Steaming is a gentle and slow-cooking method that helps to preserve the natural flavors and nutrients of the food. In TCM, steaming is considered to be a neutral cooking technique that does not add any warming or cooling properties to the food. Steaming is a good option for those who are looking to maintain their body's balance.

Boiling is another common cooking technique in TCM nutrition. Boiling is considered to be a cooling cooking method that helps to clear heat from the body. This is especially important during the hot summer months when the body tends to be overheated. Boiling is also a good option for those who have a tendency to be too warm or are experiencing symptoms of heat-related conditions.

Stir-frying is a popular cooking technique that is widely used in Chinese cuisine. Stir-frying is a quick cooking method that involves cooking small pieces of food over high heat with a small amount of oil. Stir-frying is considered to be a warming cooking technique that helps to invigorate the body's energy. This technique is especially beneficial for those who are feeling cold or experiencing symptoms of cold-related conditions.

Baking is a dry heat cooking method that is commonly used for bread and pastry making. In TCM nutrition, baking is considered to be a warming cooking method that helps to strengthen the digestive system. Baked foods are often considered to be heavy and nourishing, and they are best consumed during the winter months when the body needs more nourishment.

Roasting is a dry heat cooking method that is similar to baking. Roasting is considered to be a warming cooking method that helps to strengthen the digestive system and nourish the body. Roasted foods are often considered to be heavy and nourishing, and they are best consumed during the winter months.

In addition to the cooking techniques mentioned above, TCM nutrition also emphasizes the importance of using the right cooking equipment. In TCM, it is believed that certain materials can affect the energy properties of the food. For example, it is recommended to use clay pots for boiling and steaming, as clay is believed to add a neutral energy to the food. Stainless steel and cast iron cookware are also considered to be good options for TCM cooking.

When choosing the right cooking technique for achieving balance, it is important to consider the individual's constitution and any health conditions that they may have. For example, a person who is experiencing symptoms of heat-related conditions should avoid warming cooking techniques like stir-frying and roasting, and instead opt for cooling cooking techniques like boiling and steaming. Similarly, a person who is feeling cold should avoid cooling cooking techniques like boiling, and instead opt for warming cooking techniques like stir-frying and roasting.

Chapter Nineteen

Planning Balanced TCM Meals

In Traditional Chinese Medicine (TCM) nutrition, meal planning is essential for achieving and maintaining balance in the body. A balanced TCM meal includes a variety of food groups and flavors that work together to support overall health and wellbeing. Below we will explore some key principles for planning balanced TCM meals.

One of the main principles of TCM nutrition is the concept of the Five Elements. The Five Elements are Wood, Fire, Earth, Metal, and Water, and each element corresponds to a specific organ system in the body. To support the balance of the Five Elements, a TCM meal should include a variety of flavors and food groups. These food groups are sour, bitter, sweet, spicy, and salty, and they correspond to the Five Elements as follows:

Sour foods correspond to the Wood element and the liver and gallbladder organ systems.

Bitter foods correspond to the Fire element and the heart and small intestine organ systems.

Sweet foods correspond to the Earth element and the spleen and stomach organ systems.

Spicy foods correspond to the Metal element and the lung and large intestine organ systems.

Salty foods correspond to the Water element and the kidney and bladder organ systems.

To create a balanced TCM meal, it is important to include a variety of flavors and food groups that correspond to the different organ systems. For example, a TCM meal might include a sour dish to support the liver and gallbladder, a bitter dish to support the heart and small intestine, a sweet dish to support the spleen and stomach, a spicy dish to support the lung and large intestine, and a salty dish to support the kidney and bladder.

Another key principle of TCM nutrition is the concept of Yin and Yang. Yin and Yang are opposing but complementary forces that exist in all things. In the context of food, Yin foods are cooling, moistening, and nourishing, while Yang foods are warming, drying, and energizing. To create a balanced TCM meal, it is important to include both Yin and Yang foods. This might mean including some cooling, Yin foods like fruits and vegetables alongside warming, Yang foods like meats and grains.

In addition to including a variety of flavors and food groups, it is important to consider the cooking methods used to prepare the meal. In TCM nutrition, certain cooking methods are believed to be better suited to certain food groups and flavors. For example, steaming is considered a gentle cooking method that helps to preserve the natural moisture and flavor of the food. Steaming is often recommended for cooking vegetables, as it helps to retain their nutritional value. Stir-frying, on the other hand, is a more vigorous cooking method that can be used for heartier ingredients like meats and grains. Stir-frying can help to enhance the flavor of the food and promote digestion.

When planning a TCM meal, it is also important to consider the timing and frequency of meals. In TCM, it is recommended to eat three meals a day, with breakfast being the most important meal. Eating a substantial breakfast can help to support digestion and energy throughout the day. It is also important to avoid snacking between meals, as this can disrupt the digestive process.

Finally, it is important to pay attention to the quality and sourcing of ingredients when planning a TCM meal. Whenever possible, choose fresh, whole foods that are locally sourced and in season. This helps to ensure that the food is at its peak nutrition and flavor. It is also important to avoid processed foods and artificial ingredients, as these can disrupt the balance of the body.

Creating a balanced meal plan

1. Creating a Balanced Meal Plan: A Guide to TCM Nutrition

Food plays a crucial role in Traditional Chinese Medicine (TCM) in maintaining optimal health and preventing illness. TCM focuses on the concept of balance, which includes balancing the body's energies and balancing the nutritional content of meals. A balanced meal plan includes a variety of foods that provide the necessary nutrients to support overall health. In this article, we will discuss how to create a balanced meal plan according to TCM principles.

The Five Elements and TCM Nutrition

2. TCM believes that everything in the universe is interconnected and can be categorized into five elements: wood, fire, earth, metal, and water. Each element corresponds to a specific organ system in the body, and each organ system has different nutritional requirements.

For example, the wood element corresponds to the liver and gallbladder, and foods that are sour and green are beneficial for this element. The fire element corresponds to the heart and small intestine, and foods that are bitter and red are beneficial. The earth element corresponds to the stomach and spleen, and foods that are sweet and yellow are beneficial. The metal element corresponds to the lungs and large intestine, and foods that are pungent and white are beneficial. The water element corresponds to the kidneys and bladder, and foods that are salty and black are beneficial.

To create a balanced meal plan, it is important to include foods from each element. This ensures that all the organ systems in the body receive the nutrients they need to function optimally.

The Importance of Yin and Yang

TCM also emphasizes the importance of balancing yin and yang energies in the body. Yin represents cooling and calming energy, while yang represents warming and active energy. Both yin and yang are necessary for optimal health, and an imbalance in either can lead to illness.

Foods are categorized as yin or yang based on their energetic properties. For example, cooling foods like cucumber and watermelon are considered yin, while warming foods like ginger and cinnamon are considered yang. A balanced meal plan includes a variety of yin and yang foods to maintain optimal health.

TCM Nutrition Guidelines for a Balanced Meal Plan

In addition to considering the five elements and yin and yang energies, there are some general guidelines to follow when creating a balanced meal plan according to TCM principles. Here are some tips to keep in mind:

Variety is key. A balanced meal plan should include a variety of foods from all five elements to ensure that all organ systems are supported.

Focus on whole foods. Processed and refined foods should be avoided as much as possible, as they do not provide the same nutritional benefits as whole foods.

Pay attention to cooking methods. Different cooking methods can impact the energetic properties of foods. Steaming and stir-frying are considered healthier cooking methods in TCM.

Eat in moderation. Overeating can lead to imbalances in the body. Eating slowly and mindfully can help prevent overeating.

Stay hydrated. Drinking plenty of water and herbal teas can help support the body's natural detoxification processes.

Sample Balanced Meal Plan

Here is an example of a balanced meal plan according to TCM principles:

3. Breakfast: A bowl of oatmeal with sliced banana, walnuts, and a drizzle of honey. This provides a combination of sweet and neutral flavors and includes elements from wood, earth, and water.

4. Lunch: A stir-fry with chicken, broccoli, carrots, and bell peppers served over brown rice. This provides a combination of sweet, sour, and bitter flavors and includes elements from wood, earth, and metal.

5. Snack: Sliced cucumber and hummus. This provides a cooling and calming snack that is yin in nature.

6. Dinner: Baked salmon with roasted sweet potatoes and Brussels spr

TCM meal planning tips and ideas

Traditional Chinese Medicine (TCM) emphasizes the importance of a balanced and wholesome diet for optimal health and well-being. In TCM, food is considered medicine, and a well-planned meal can help restore balance and promote vitality. However, with the vast array of food options available, it can be overwhelming to determine what to eat and how to create a balanced meal plan. Here are some TCM meal planning tips and ideas to help you get started.

Follow the Five-Element Theory

1. TCM is based on the Five-Element Theory, which categorizes food into five groups: wood, fire, earth, metal, and water. Each element corresponds to a specific organ and has different nutritional properties. A balanced meal plan should include all five elements in appropriate proportions to promote overall balance and health.

For example, a meal that includes leafy greens (wood element) for the liver, brown rice (earth element) for the spleen, chicken (metal element) for the lungs, tomatoes (fire element) for the heart, and tofu (water element) for the kidneys would create a balanced and wholesome meal.

Consider Yin-Yang Balance

TCM also emphasizes the importance of yin-yang balance in food. Yin and yang are opposite but complementary forces that exist in all things, including food. Yin foods are cool and moist, while yang foods are warm and dry. A balanced meal plan should include a variety of yin and yang foods in appropriate proportions to promote overall balance and health.

For example, a meal that includes steamed fish (yin) with ginger (yang) and vegetables stir-fried with sesame oil (yang) and soy sauce (yin) would create a balanced and wholesome meal.

Include a Variety of Colors

In TCM, each color represents a different nutrient and has specific health benefits. A meal plan that includes a variety of colors can help ensure that you are getting a range of nutrients and promoting overall health and well-being.

For example, a meal that includes red peppers (vitamin C and antioxidants), sweet potatoes (vitamin A and fiber), broccoli (vitamin K and calcium), blueberries (antioxidants), and black beans (fiber and protein) would create a colorful and nutrient-dense meal.

Eat Seasonally and Locally

TCM emphasizes the importance of eating seasonally and locally. Eating foods that are in season and grown locally can help ensure that you are getting fresh and nutrient-dense foods. In addition, seasonal and local foods are believed to be more energetically aligned with the body's needs, promoting overall health and balance.

For example, in the summer, a meal that includes watermelon (cooling and hydrating), cucumber (cooling and detoxifying), tomatoes (cooling and nourishing), and grilled corn (warming and grounding) would create a balanced and seasonally appropriate meal.

Use Herbs and Spices for Flavor and Health Benefits

Herbs and spices not only add flavor to food but also have specific health benefits. In TCM, herbs and spices are used for their medicinal properties and can help promote overall health and well-being.

For example, adding ginger to a stir-fry can help improve digestion and reduce inflammation. Adding turmeric to a curry can help boost the immune system and reduce inflammation. Adding cinnamon to oatmeal can help regulate blood sugar levels and improve circulation.

Chapter Twenty

TCM Nutrition Recipes

Traditional Chinese Medicine (TCM) nutrition is an important aspect of health and wellness. It focuses on the use of food to maintain balance and harmony within the body. TCM practitioners believe that different foods have different energetic properties that can affect the body's Qi, or life force energy. Therefore, a balanced TCM diet is one that includes a variety of foods that support and nourish the body.

Here are some TCM nutrition recipes that are easy to make and can be incorporated into a healthy and balanced diet:

Congee

Congee is a type of rice porridge that is commonly eaten in Asian countries. It is a staple in TCM nutrition as it is easy to digest and provides a good source of energy. Congee can be made with various ingredients such as vegetables, meat, and herbs, depending on the individual's needs. Here is a simple recipe for congee:

Ingredients:

1 cup of rice

6 cups of water or broth

1-inch piece of ginger, sliced

2 garlic cloves, minced

Salt and pepper to taste

1. Optional toppings: sliced scallions, chopped cilantro, sesame oil, soy sauce

Instructions:

Rinse the rice and place it in a pot with the water or broth.

Add the ginger and garlic to the pot and bring to a boil.

Reduce heat to low and simmer for 1-2 hours, stirring occasionally, until the rice has broken down and the mixture is thick and creamy.

Season with salt and pepper to taste.

Serve hot with desired toppings.

Steamed Fish with Ginger and Scallions

This dish is a classic in TCM nutrition as it is believed to nourish the blood and improve circulation. It is also low in fat and calories, making it a healthy and nutritious option.

Ingredients:

1 whole fish (such as sea bass or red snapper), cleaned and scaled

2-inch piece of ginger, sliced

2 scallions, sliced

2 tbsp of soy sauce

1 tbsp of rice wine

1 tbsp of sesame oil

Salt and pepper to taste

Instructions:

Place the fish on a heatproof plate and season with salt and pepper.

Top the fish with the ginger and scallions.

In a separate bowl, mix together the soy sauce, rice wine, and sesame oil. Pour the mixture over the fish.

Steam the fish for about 15-20 minutes or until cooked through.

Serve hot with steamed rice.

Stir-Fried Vegetables with Tofu

This recipe is a great way to incorporate more vegetables into your diet. Tofu is a good source of protein and the vegetables provide fiber and nutrients.

Ingredients:

1 block of tofu, cubed

2 cups of mixed vegetables (such as broccoli, carrots, bell peppers, and mushrooms), sliced

2 garlic cloves, minced

1-inch piece of ginger, grated

2 tbsp of soy sauce

1 tbsp of honey

1 tbsp of sesame oil

Salt and pepper to taste

Instructions:

Heat a wok or large skillet over high heat.

Add the tofu and stir-fry for 2-3 minutes until lightly browned. Remove from pan and set aside.

Add the vegetables to the pan and stir-fry for 2-3 minutes until crisp-tender.

Add the garlic and ginger to the pan and stir-fry for another minute.

In a small bowl, mix together the soy sauce, honey, and sesame oil. Pour the mixture over the

Breakfast recipes

Breakfast is the most important meal of the day, as it sets the tone for your energy and mood for the rest of the day. In Traditional Chinese Medicine (TCM), breakfast is considered as a crucial meal that can support the body's natural rhythms and balance. Eating a nutritious breakfast can help to strengthen digestion, support mental clarity, and promote vitality. Below we will explore some TCM breakfast recipes that can provide the necessary nutrition for a healthy start to the day.

Congee

Congee, also known as rice porridge, is a popular breakfast dish in China. It is a simple and easy-to-digest meal that is perfect for those with weak digestive systems. Congee can be made with various grains such as rice, millet, or quinoa, and can be flavored with a range of vegetables and spices. To prepare congee, use one cup of grain to six cups of water, and cook on low heat until the grains are soft and creamy. Add chopped vegetables such as carrots, onions, and mushrooms, and season with ginger, garlic, and soy sauce for added flavor.

Oatmeal with nuts and berries

Oatmeal is a classic breakfast dish that is packed with nutrients and fiber. In TCM, oats are believed to strengthen the digestive system, regulate blood sugar levels, and nourish the Yin energy in the body. To prepare oatmeal, cook rolled oats in water or milk, and add a handful of chopped nuts such as almonds or walnuts, and fresh or frozen berries such as blueberries or raspberries. You can also add a dash of cinnamon or honey for added sweetness.

Steamed eggs with vegetables

Steamed eggs with vegetables is a quick and easy breakfast dish that is rich in protein and essential vitamins. To prepare, beat two eggs in a bowl, and add chopped vegetables such as spinach, kale, or bell peppers. Pour the mixture into a heatproof bowl, and steam for about 10-15 minutes, or until the eggs are set. Season with salt and pepper to taste.

Smoothie bowl

Smoothie bowls are a delicious and nutritious breakfast option that is perfect for those on-the-go. To make a smoothie bowl, blend a variety of fruits and vegetables such as bananas, berries, kale, spinach, and almond milk. Pour the mixture into a bowl, and top with nuts, seeds, and granola for added crunch and texture.

Rice cakes with avocado and smoked salmon

Rice cakes with avocado and smoked salmon is a savory and satisfying breakfast dish that is perfect for those who prefer a heartier meal. To prepare, toast rice cakes, and top with mashed avocado, smoked salmon, and sliced cucumber. Season with salt and pepper to taste, and garnish with fresh herbs such as cilantro or parsley.

Lunch recipes

In Traditional Chinese Medicine (TCM), lunch is considered the most important meal of the day. It is believed that eating a balanced, nutritious lunch can provide the energy and nourishment necessary for the body to function properly throughout the day. Below we will discuss some TCM-inspired lunch recipes that are both delicious and healthful.

Congee with Vegetables

Congee is a traditional Chinese rice porridge that is commonly eaten for breakfast, but it can also be enjoyed as a hearty and warming lunch. To make congee, simply cook one cup of rice in six cups of water until the rice is completely broken down and the mixture has a porridge-like consistency. Add any vegetables you like, such as carrots, broccoli, and kale, and season with ginger, garlic, and a touch of soy sauce. This dish is easy to digest and can help to soothe the stomach and nourish the digestive system.

Stir-Fry with Tofu and Vegetables

Stir-fries are a popular lunch option in TCM, as they are easy to prepare and can be customized to include a variety of vegetables and proteins. To make a stir-fry with tofu and vegetables, heat a tablespoon of oil in a wok or frying pan and add thinly sliced tofu. Cook until the tofu is golden brown, then remove from the pan and set aside. Add sliced vegetables, such as bell peppers, broccoli, and mushrooms, and cook until tender. Season with garlic, ginger, and a touch of soy sauce, then add the tofu back to the pan and stir to combine. Serve over brown rice or quinoa for a complete meal.

Miso Soup with Soba Noodles

Miso soup is a popular Japanese dish that is also commonly enjoyed in TCM. To make miso soup, simply heat water in a pot and add a tablespoon of miso paste. Stir until the miso is dissolved, then add sliced mushrooms, diced tofu, and cooked soba noodles. Bring to a boil and simmer for a few minutes until the mushrooms are tender and the noodles are heated through. Season with a touch of soy sauce and sliced green onions for added flavor.

Steamed Fish with Vegetables

In TCM, steaming is considered one of the healthiest cooking methods, as it helps to preserve the nutrients in food. To make steamed fish with vegetables, simply season a fillet of fish with ginger, garlic, and soy sauce, then place it on a plate with sliced vegetables, such as bok choy and carrots. Steam for 10-15 minutes until the fish is cooked through and the vegetables are tender. Serve with a side of brown rice or quinoa for a complete meal.

Buddha Bowl with Brown Rice and Vegetables

Buddha bowls are a trendy and nutritious lunch option that can be customized to include a variety of vegetables and proteins. To make a TCM-inspired Buddha bowl, start with a base of cooked brown rice and add a variety of vegetables, such as kale, spinach, and roasted sweet potatoes. Top with sliced avocado, sliced almonds, and a protein of your choice, such as grilled chicken or tofu. Drizzle with a homemade dressing made from olive oil, lemon juice, and a touch of honey.

Dinner recipes

Dinner is often considered the most important meal of the day, as it is typically the last meal before a long period of rest and fasting during sleep. In

Traditional Chinese Medicine (TCM), dinner is also an important time for nourishing the body with foods that support balance and health. Below we will explore some TCM-inspired dinner recipes that incorporate a variety of nutrient-rich ingredients to support optimal health and well-being.

TCM Chicken and Mushroom Stir Fry

Ingredients:

1 pound boneless, skinless chicken breasts, sliced thin

1 cup sliced mushrooms

1 cup chopped bok choy

1 cup sliced carrots

1 tablespoon grated ginger

2 cloves garlic, minced

2 tablespoons soy sauce

2 tablespoons hoisin sauce

1 tablespoon rice vinegar

1 tablespoon cornstarch

2 tablespoons vegetable oil

Instructions:

In a small bowl, whisk together the soy sauce, hoisin sauce, rice vinegar, and cornstarch until smooth.

In a large skillet or wok, heat the vegetable oil over high heat. Add the chicken and stir-fry until browned and cooked through, about 5-7 minutes.

Add the mushrooms, bok choy, carrots, ginger, and garlic to the skillet and stir-fry for an additional 3-5 minutes, until the vegetables are tender.

Pour the sauce over the chicken and vegetables and stir-fry for 1-2 minutes, until the sauce has thickened and coated the ingredients evenly.

Serve hot over rice or noodles.

This stir fry recipe is a great way to incorporate a variety of TCM ingredients into your dinner. Chicken is a good source of protein, while mushrooms are known to support the immune system and promote healthy digestion. Bok choy is a nutrient-dense vegetable that is rich in vitamins and minerals, while ginger and garlic have anti-inflammatory properties that may help reduce inflammation in the body.

TCM Salmon and Quinoa Bowl

Ingredients:

1 pound salmon fillet

1 cup cooked quinoa

1 cup chopped kale

1 cup sliced bell peppers

1/2 cup chopped scallions

1/4 cup soy sauce

2 tablespoons honey

1 tablespoon rice vinegar

1 tablespoon sesame oil

1 tablespoon grated ginger

2 cloves garlic, minced

Salt and pepper to taste

Instructions:

Preheat the oven to 375°F.

Season the salmon fillet with salt and pepper and place it on a baking sheet lined with parchment paper. Bake for 15-20 minutes, until cooked through.

In a small bowl, whisk together the soy sauce, honey, rice vinegar, sesame oil, ginger, and garlic until well combined.

In a large skillet or wok, heat a tablespoon of vegetable oil over medium-high heat. Add the kale and bell peppers and stir-fry for 2-3 minutes, until the vegetables are slightly softened.

Add the cooked quinoa to the skillet and stir-fry for an additional 2-3 minutes, until the quinoa is heated through and slightly crispy.

Pour the sauce over the quinoa and vegetables and stir-fry for 1-2 minutes, until the ingredients are coated evenly.

Serve the salmon fillet over the quinoa and vegetable mixture, and garnish with chopped scallions.

This salmon and quinoa bowl is a nutrient-dense dinner that is rich in omega-3 fatty acids, protein, and fiber. Salmon is known to support heart health and cognitive function

Snack and dessert recipes

TCM nutrition emphasizes the importance of balancing the energy and nourishment of the body through food. This ancient practice is centered around the belief that food can be used as medicine to prevent and treat illnesses. In TCM, snacks and desserts are not just indulgent treats, but can also be a part of a balanced diet that supports optimal health.

When it comes to snacks, TCM recommends choosing foods that are high in protein and complex carbohydrates to help sustain energy and prevent blood sugar spikes. Some great options include roasted chickpeas, edamame, raw vegetables with hummus, and whole grain crackers with nut butter.

In addition to snacks, TCM also recognizes the importance of incorporating sweet flavors into the diet, but in a balanced way that doesn't disrupt the body's energy flow. One way to do this is by incorporating natural sweeteners such as honey, maple syrup, and dates into desserts.

Here are three TCM-inspired snack and dessert recipes:

Roasted Chickpeas

Roasted chickpeas are a great snack option that are high in protein and fiber. They also have a satisfying crunch that makes them a great substitute for unhealthy snacks like chips.

Ingredients:

1 can of chickpeas, drained and rinsed

1 tablespoon of olive oil

1 teaspoon of cumin

1 teaspoon of paprika

1/2 teaspoon of garlic powder

Salt and pepper to taste

Instructions:

Preheat oven to 400°F.

Spread the chickpeas out on a baking sheet and drizzle with olive oil.

Sprinkle the spices over the chickpeas and toss to coat.

Roast in the oven for 20-25 minutes or until crispy, shaking the pan occasionally to prevent burning.

Honey-Sweetened Granola Bars

These granola bars are a great option for a quick and easy snack that's packed with protein and fiber. They also have the perfect balance of sweet and salty flavors.

Ingredients:

2 cups of rolled oats

1/2 cup of almonds, chopped

1/2 cup of dried cranberries

1/4 cup of honey

1/4 cup of coconut oil

1/4 teaspoon of salt

Instructions:

Preheat oven to 350°F.

In a large bowl, mix together the oats, almonds, and cranberries.

In a small saucepan, heat the honey, coconut oil, and salt over low heat until melted and combined.

Pour the honey mixture over the oat mixture and stir to combine.

Press the mixture into an 8x8 inch baking dish lined with parchment paper.

Bake for 25-30 minutes or until golden brown.

Let cool completely before cutting into bars.

Baked Pears with Cinnamon and Dates

This simple dessert is a great way to satisfy a sweet tooth while also incorporating fruit and natural sweeteners.

Ingredients:

2 pears, halved and cored

4 dates, chopped

1 teaspoon of cinnamon

2 tablespoons of honey

2 tablespoons of water

Instructions:

Preheat oven to 375°F.

Place the pear halves in a baking dish.

In a small bowl, mix together the dates and cinnamon.

Stuff the date mixture into the center of the pear halves.

Drizzle the honey and water over the pears.

Bake for 25-30 minutes or until the pears are soft and caramelized.

Chapter Twenty-One

Integrating TCM Nutrition into Daily Life

Traditional Chinese Medicine (TCM) has been a cornerstone of health and wellness in China for thousands of years. It is an ancient system of healing that aims to restore balance and harmony to the body, mind, and spirit. TCM encompasses various modalities, including acupuncture, herbal medicine, and dietary therapy. TCM dietary therapy emphasizes the concept of food as medicine and focuses on using food to prevent and treat illnesses. It is believed that a balanced diet can promote good health, prevent disease, and help the body heal. Below we will explore some practical tips on integrating TCM nutrition into daily life.

Start with the basics

TCM nutrition emphasizes eating whole foods that are fresh, locally grown, and in season. This means avoiding processed foods, refined sugars, and unhealthy fats. Whole grains, vegetables, fruits, legumes, and lean proteins should make up the bulk of the diet. In TCM, each food has its own unique properties, which can be used to address specific health concerns. For example, ginger is considered warming and can be used to alleviate colds and digestive issues. Garlic is considered pungent and can help to prevent cardiovascular disease. By incorporating a variety of whole foods into the diet, individuals can benefit from their unique health properties.

Understand your body constitution

1. According to TCM, everyone has a unique body constitution based on their individual genetics and life experiences. Understanding one's constitution is crucial to achieving optimal health. There are five primary constitutions in TCM: Wood, Fire, Earth, Metal, and Water. Each constitution has unique characteristics and dietary needs. For example, individuals with a Wood constitution tend to have a high metabolism and benefit from cooling foods, such as cucumbers and watermelon. Individuals with a Fire constitution tend to have a tendency towards inflammation and benefit from anti-inflammatory foods, such as turmeric and ginger. By understanding one's constitution, individuals can tailor their diet to their specific needs.

Incorporate TCM herbs and spices

Herbs and spices play a significant role in TCM nutrition. They can be used to add flavor to meals and provide numerous health benefits. For example, cinnamon is considered warming and can help to regulate blood sugar levels. Turmeric is considered anti-inflammatory and can help to reduce inflammation in the body. Ginger is considered warming and can help to alleviate nausea and digestive issues. By incorporating these herbs and spices into meals, individuals can benefit from their health-promoting properties.

Practice mindful eating

Mindful eating is a fundamental principle in TCM nutrition. It involves being fully present and aware during meals, focusing on the taste, texture, and aroma of the food. Mindful eating can help to improve digestion, prevent overeating, and promote a sense of satisfaction after meals. It is also important to eat in a relaxed environment, away from distractions such as phones and computers. By practicing mindful eating, individuals can develop a deeper connection with their food and promote optimal digestion and absorption of nutrients.

Cook at home

Cooking at home is one of the best ways to integrate TCM nutrition into daily life. Home-cooked meals are typically healthier and more nutrient-dense than restaurant or fast food meals. By cooking at home, individuals can control the ingredients, portion sizes, and cooking methods used in their meals. This can help to ensure that meals are balanced and tailored to their specific needs. Additionally, cooking at home can be a fun and rewarding experience that promotes creativity and experimentation in the kitchen.

Seek guidance from a TCM practitioner

Integrating TCM nutrition into daily life can be a complex process, especially for those new to the concept. Seeking guidance from a qualified TCM practitioner can be beneficial in developing a personalized dietary plan that meets individual needs. A T

Tips for implementing TCM nutrition principles

Traditional Chinese Medicine (TCM) nutrition principles offer a holistic approach to eating that considers not just the nutritional value of food but also its energetic properties and how it affects the body's organs and systems. Integrating TCM nutrition into daily life may seem overwhelming at first, but with some simple tips and guidelines, it can become a natural and intuitive part of your lifestyle.

Start with small changes

Integrating TCM nutrition principles into your diet doesn't have to mean a complete overhaul of your eating habits. Start with small changes, such as incorporating more whole foods, seasonal produce, and healthy cooking techniques into your meals. Gradually incorporate more TCM principles over time to make it a sustainable and lasting lifestyle change.

Emphasize balance and moderation

TCM nutrition emphasizes the importance of balance and moderation in food choices. Rather than following strict rules or diets, focus on including a variety of whole foods, including grains, vegetables, fruits, protein sources, and healthy fats, in appropriate portions. Listen to your body and adjust your portions and food choices accordingly.

Eat seasonally

In TCM, the body is viewed as part of the natural world and influenced by the seasons. Eating seasonally helps to nourish and support the body in each season's unique energy. Focus on including seasonal fruits and vegetables in your meals and adjusting your diet to suit the needs of your body and the environment.

Consider food energetics

TCM nutrition principles recognize that food has energetic properties that can affect the body's organs and systems. Foods are categorized as cooling, warming, damp, or dry, and each category has a unique effect on the body. For example, warming foods are thought to increase circulation and energy, while cooling foods are thought to reduce inflammation and heat in the body. Consider incorporating a balance of cooling and warming foods in your diet to support the body's overall balance.

Choose healthy cooking techniques

The way you cook your food can impact its nutritional value and energetic properties. TCM emphasizes cooking techniques that preserve the food's nutrients and energetic properties, such as steaming, boiling, and stir-frying. Avoid cooking methods that involve high heat or deep-frying, which can destroy nutrients and create harmful byproducts.

Pay attention to food combinations

In TCM, food combinations are thought to impact digestion and nutrient absorption. For example, combining foods with conflicting energetics or improper proportions can disrupt digestion and lead to bloating and other digestive issues. Aim to combine foods that complement each other and promote healthy digestion.

Mindful eating

TCM nutrition also emphasizes the importance of mindful eating, which involves paying attention to the food's taste, texture, and how it affects the body. By slowing down and savoring each bite, you can improve digestion, reduce stress, and enhance the overall eating experience.

Seek guidance from a qualified practitioner

While these tips can help you integrate TCM nutrition principles into your daily life, seeking guidance from a qualified TCM practitioner can provide personalized advice and recommendations. A practitioner can help you identify your body's unique needs and recommend specific foods, herbs, and supplements to support your health and well-being.

Cultivating mindfulness around food and eating

Cultivating mindfulness around food and eating is an important aspect of Traditional Chinese Medicine (TCM) nutrition. In TCM, the focus is not just on what you eat, but also on how you eat, and the intention and mindset that you bring to your meals. Mindful eating practices can help to improve digestion, reduce stress, and enhance overall well-being.

One of the key principles of TCM nutrition is that every person is unique and has individual needs. This means that there is no one-size-fits-all approach to eating. In order to determine the best approach for you, it is important to first understand your body type and the imbalances that you may be experiencing. This can be done through a TCM consultation with a qualified practitioner, who can provide personalized dietary recommendations.

Once you have an understanding of your individual needs, it is important to approach food with a sense of mindfulness and intention. This means taking the time to prepare and savor your meals, rather than rushing through them or eating on the go. It also means being present and fully engaged in the act of eating, rather than being distracted by technology, work, or other stressors.

Another aspect of mindfulness around food is paying attention to how different foods affect your body. TCM emphasizes the importance of eating foods that are in season and that are appropriate for your individual constitution. This means that some foods may be beneficial for one person, but not for another. By paying attention to how your body responds to different foods, you can make more informed choices about what to eat.

In addition to mindfulness around food, TCM also emphasizes the importance of proper food preparation and cooking techniques. In TCM, the goal is to maximize the nutritional value of foods and to ensure that they are easy to digest. This may involve using specific cooking methods, such as steaming, boiling, or stir-frying, as well as incorporating certain herbs and spices into meals.

One technique that can help to cultivate mindfulness around food is the practice of gratitude. This involves expressing appreciation for the food that you are about to eat, as well as for the people and resources that made it possible. By cultivating a sense of gratitude and respect for food, you can develop a deeper appreciation for the nourishment that it provides and approach eating with a greater sense of reverence.

Another important aspect of mindful eating is paying attention to hunger and fullness cues. In TCM, it is believed that the body has a natural intelligence when it comes to regulating food intake. By paying attention to feelings of hunger and fullness, you can avoid overeating and ensure that you are providing your body with the nutrients that it needs without overwhelming the digestive system.

Incorporating mindfulness into your eating habits may take some practice, but there are several techniques that can help. One simple practice is to take a few deep breaths before eating, which can help to calm the mind and set a positive intention for the meal. Another technique is to eat slowly and intentionally, savoring each bite and focusing on the flavors and textures of the food.

Chapter Twenty-Two

TCM Nutrition for Detoxification and Cleansing

Traditional Chinese Medicine (TCM) is an ancient holistic system that aims to restore balance and harmony within the body through various methods, including nutrition. One aspect of TCM nutrition is detoxification and cleansing, which is an essential part of maintaining good health. Below we will explore the principles of TCM nutrition for detoxification and cleansing, including the foods to incorporate into the diet and the benefits they offer.

The Principles of TCM Nutrition for Detoxification and Cleansing

According to TCM, the body naturally eliminates toxins through various channels, including the liver, kidneys, lungs, and skin. However, when these organs become overwhelmed with toxins, it can lead to imbalances and health problems. Therefore, TCM emphasizes the importance of supporting the body's natural detoxification processes through diet and lifestyle modifications.

One of the essential principles of TCM nutrition for detoxification is the inclusion of foods that promote circulation and eliminate stagnation. These foods can help to enhance the body's ability to remove toxins and waste products, improving overall health and vitality. Additionally, TCM emphasizes the importance of consuming foods that are easy to digest, as poor digestion can lead to the accumulation of toxins in the body.

Foods for Detoxification and Cleansing

Many foods are beneficial for detoxification and cleansing in TCM nutrition. Here are some examples:

Leafy greens - Leafy greens are an excellent source of chlorophyll, a potent detoxifier. They also contain antioxidants, vitamins, and minerals that support liver function and promote circulation.

Cruciferous vegetables - Cruciferous vegetables such as broccoli, cauliflower, and cabbage contain sulfur compounds that support liver function and aid in the elimination of toxins.

Citrus fruits - Citrus fruits are high in vitamin C, a powerful antioxidant that supports the immune system and promotes detoxification.

Berries - Berries are rich in antioxidants, which help to neutralize free radicals and protect the body from oxidative stress. They are also a good source of fiber, which aids in digestion and elimination.

Turmeric - Turmeric is a potent anti-inflammatory and antioxidant that supports liver function and aids in the elimination of toxins.

Ginger - Ginger is a warming herb that promotes circulation and aids in digestion, making it an excellent choice for detoxification and cleansing.

Garlic - Garlic is a natural antibiotic and immune booster that supports liver function and aids in the elimination of toxins.

Green tea - Green tea contains antioxidants called catechins, which help to promote detoxification and reduce inflammation.

Seaweed - Seaweed is a rich source of minerals and iodine, which support thyroid function and aid in the elimination of toxins.

Mushrooms - Certain mushrooms, such as shiitake and maitake, contain compounds that support liver function and aid in the elimination of toxins.

Benefits of TCM Nutrition for Detoxification and Cleansing

Incorporating TCM nutrition principles into the diet can have numerous benefits for detoxification and cleansing, including:

Improved liver function - Many of the foods recommended for detoxification and cleansing in TCM nutrition support liver function, which is essential for eliminating toxins from the body.

Enhanced digestion - Consuming foods that are easy to digest can help to reduce the accumulation of toxins in the body and promote regular elimination.

Increased energy - When the body is free from toxins and waste products, it can function more efficiently, leading to increased energy and vitality.

Reduced inflammation - Many of the foods recommended for detoxification and cleansing in TCM nutrition are anti-inflammatory, which can help to reduce inflammation in the body and improve overall health.

Improved immune function - TCM nutrition emphasizes the importance of supporting the immune system, which

The role of detoxification in TCM

Traditional Chinese Medicine (TCM) views the body as a complex system that is affected by both internal and external factors. The food we eat, the air we breathe, and the activities we engage in all have an impact on our health. When our bodies are overwhelmed by toxins, it can lead to a wide range of health issues. TCM believes that detoxification is an essential part of maintaining overall health and well-being.

According to TCM principles, toxins accumulate in the body over time, disrupting the flow of Qi (energy) and causing imbalances. Toxins can enter our body through various sources, including processed foods, pollution, medications, alcohol, and even negative emotions. TCM emphasizes that detoxification should be a natural and ongoing process. Therefore, it is essential to incorporate TCM nutrition and dietary strategies to support the body's natural detoxification processes.

TCM nutrition for detoxification and cleansing focuses on the use of whole, natural foods that help to eliminate toxins, nourish the body, and support the organs involved in the detoxification process. One of the primary TCM organs involved in detoxification is the liver. The liver is responsible for filtering toxins from the blood and breaking them down so that they can be eliminated from the body. Therefore, it is essential to focus on foods that support the liver and help it to function properly.

Some of the best TCM foods for liver health and detoxification include bitter greens, such as kale, collard greens, and dandelion greens. These greens contain compounds that help to stimulate the liver and increase bile flow, which aids in the digestion of fats and the elimination of toxins. Other TCM foods that support liver health include beets, carrots, ginger, and garlic.

In addition to supporting liver health, TCM also emphasizes the importance of supporting the digestive system for optimal detoxification. This means incorporating foods that are high in fiber, such as whole grains, legumes, and vegetables. Fiber helps to promote bowel movements and eliminate waste from the body. It is also important to consume foods that are high in water content, such as fruits and vegetables, to help flush out toxins.

TCM nutrition for detoxification also recommends incorporating foods that are high in antioxidants. Antioxidants are compounds that help to protect the body against free radicals, which can damage cells and contribute to disease. Foods that are high in antioxidants include berries, dark leafy greens, nuts, and seeds.

Another important aspect of TCM nutrition for detoxification is the use of herbs and spices. Herbs and spices have been used for thousands of years in TCM to support detoxification and cleanse the body. Some of the most commonly used herbs and spices for detoxification include turmeric, cumin, coriander, and fennel. These herbs and spices have anti-inflammatory and antioxidant properties that help to support the liver and other organs involved in detoxification.

When it comes to TCM nutrition for detoxification, it is important to focus on whole, natural foods and avoid processed and refined foods. Processed and refined foods can contribute to the accumulation of toxins in the body and make it more difficult for the body to eliminate them. Instead, focus on foods that are rich in nutrients and support the body's natural detoxification processes.

TCM nutrition also emphasizes the importance of mindful eating. Mindful eating means paying attention to the food we eat, savoring each bite, and being present in the moment. Mindful eating can help to reduce stress and improve digestion, both of which are essential for optimal detoxification.

Foods and herbs that support detoxification

TCM nutrition emphasizes the importance of consuming whole, nourishing foods that can support the body's natural processes, including detoxification. In Traditional Chinese Medicine (TCM), the body's detoxification system is primarily regulated by the liver, which helps to filter out toxins and waste products from the body. However, other organs such as the lungs, kidneys, and skin also play a role in the detoxification process. Below we will discuss the foods and herbs that can support and enhance the body's natural detoxification process.

One of the key principles of TCM nutrition is to eat a variety of foods in moderation. Consuming a balanced diet that includes a range of fruits, vegetables, whole grains, and lean protein sources is important for supporting overall health and well-being. When it comes to detoxification, there are several foods and herbs that can be particularly beneficial.

1. Cruciferous Vegetables: Cruciferous vegetables such as broccoli, cauliflower, and Brussels sprouts are rich in glucosinolates, compounds that can help to support the liver's detoxification pathways. These vegetables are also high in fiber, which can help to promote regular bowel movements and remove toxins from the body.

2. Leafy Greens: Leafy greens such as spinach, kale, and Swiss chard are excellent sources of antioxidants, which can help to protect the body's cells from damage caused by toxins. These greens are also rich in chlorophyll, a pigment that has been shown to support liver detoxification.

3. Garlic: Garlic is a powerful herb that has been used for centuries in TCM for its medicinal properties. Garlic contains sulfur compounds that can help to support the liver's detoxification pathways and also has anti-inflammatory properties.

4. Turmeric: Turmeric is a spice that has been used in TCM for thousands of years for its anti-inflammatory and antioxidant properties. The active

ingredient in turmeric, curcumin, has been shown to support liver detoxification and may also have anti-cancer properties.

5. Dandelion Root: Dandelion root is a common herb used in TCM to support liver detoxification. It contains compounds that can help to increase bile flow and support the liver's ability to remove toxins from the body.

6. Milk Thistle: Milk thistle is another herb commonly used in TCM to support liver health and detoxification. It contains silymarin, a compound that has been shown to protect the liver from damage and support the liver's detoxification pathways.

In addition to these foods and herbs, it is also important to stay hydrated by drinking plenty of water and consuming herbal teas such as green tea and dandelion tea. Water helps to flush toxins from the body, while herbal teas can provide additional support for the liver and other detoxification pathways.

It is also important to limit or avoid processed foods, alcohol, and other substances that can be harmful to the body. Processed foods can be high in additives, preservatives, and other chemicals that can put additional stress on the liver and other organs involved in detoxification. Alcohol can also be damaging to the liver and should be consumed in moderation or avoided altogether.

Chapter Twenty-Three

TCM Nutrition for Healthy Skin

Traditional Chinese Medicine (TCM) has a holistic approach to health that considers the interconnectedness of the mind, body, and spirit. TCM emphasizes the importance of balance and harmony in all aspects of life, including nutrition. According to TCM, the appearance and health of the skin are directly related to the health of the internal organs, particularly the lungs, spleen, and kidneys. Therefore, TCM nutrition for healthy skin involves nourishing these organs with the right foods and herbs to promote optimal functioning and balance in the body.

The lungs are responsible for circulating oxygen and removing waste products from the body. According to TCM, the skin is connected to the lungs through the pores, which are channels for waste removal. Therefore, the health of the lungs can affect the appearance and health of the skin. Foods that support lung health include those that are high in antioxidants and anti-inflammatory compounds, such as leafy greens, berries, and turmeric. These foods can help to protect the lungs from damage and promote their optimal functioning.

The spleen is responsible for digestion and the distribution of nutrients throughout the body. According to TCM, the spleen is also responsible for maintaining the body's qi (energy) and blood. When the spleen is weak or imbalanced, it can lead to skin problems such as acne, eczema, and psoriasis. Foods that support spleen health include those that are easily digestible, such as cooked vegetables, whole grains, and soups. Additionally, warming and nourishing foods such as ginger, cinnamon, and chicken can also help to support the spleen.

The kidneys are responsible for filtering waste products from the blood and regulating the body's fluid balance. According to TCM, the kidneys are also responsible for the health and vitality of the hair and nails, which are considered to be an extension of the skin. Therefore, the health of the kidneys can also affect the appearance and health of the skin. Foods that support kidney health include those that are high in minerals such as calcium, magnesium, and potassium, such as leafy greens, nuts, and seeds. Additionally, foods that are high in essential fatty acids, such as salmon and avocado, can also help to nourish the kidneys and promote healthy skin.

In addition to specific foods, there are also a number of herbs that are commonly used in TCM to support healthy skin. One of the most commonly used herbs is Schisandra, which is known for its ability to support the liver and promote healthy skin. Another herb that is commonly used in TCM is Rehmannia, which is known for its ability to nourish the blood and promote healthy skin. Other herbs that are commonly used in TCM for healthy skin include Burdock, Dandelion, and Licorice root.

When it comes to TCM nutrition for healthy skin, it is important to focus on whole, nutrient-dense foods and avoid processed and refined foods that can contribute to inflammation and oxidative stress in the body. It is also important to stay hydrated by drinking plenty of water and herbal teas. In TCM, it is believed that cold beverages and foods can weaken the spleen and impair digestion, so it is recommended to consume foods and beverages at room temperature or slightly warm.

Incorporating TCM nutrition principles into your daily life can be a simple and effective way to support healthy skin from the inside out. Some easy ways to do this include:

Start your day with warm water and lemon to support digestion and hydration.

Incorporate a variety of colorful fruits and vegetables into your meals to provide a range of nutrients and antioxidants.

Swap out processed snacks for whole foods such as nuts, seeds, and fresh fruit.

Choose warming and nourishing foods such as soups, stews

The connection between diet and skin health

The skin is the body's largest organ, and its health and appearance are often a reflection of our internal health. It is well established that diet plays a crucial role in skin health, with certain foods and nutrients being beneficial for promoting healthy, clear, and vibrant skin. Traditional Chinese Medicine (TCM) has long recognized the connection between diet and skin health and emphasizes the use of nutrition to maintain healthy skin. Below we will explore the connection between diet and skin health from a TCM perspective and discuss some of the best foods and nutrients for promoting healthy skin.

In TCM, the skin is closely related to the lungs, which are responsible for circulating oxygen and energy throughout the body. When the lungs are functioning well, the skin is nourished with oxygen and nutrients, resulting in healthy and glowing skin. However, when the lungs are not functioning correctly, the skin can become dry, dull, and prone to wrinkles and blemishes.

One of the key principles of TCM nutrition for healthy skin is to eat foods that promote proper lung function. This includes foods that are rich in antioxidants, such as fruits and vegetables, which help to protect the lungs and other organs from oxidative stress. In addition, TCM emphasizes the importance of eating foods that are rich in qi (pronounced "chee"), the vital energy that is essential for good health. Foods that are rich in qi include whole grains, beans, nuts, and seeds, which provide sustained energy and support overall health and vitality.

Another important aspect of TCM nutrition for healthy skin is to eat foods that are rich in moisture. In TCM, dry skin is often seen as a sign of an imbalance in the body, and eating foods that help to moisten the body can be beneficial for promoting healthy skin. This includes foods that are high in water content, such as fruits and vegetables, as well as foods that contain healthy fats, such as avocados and nuts.

In addition to eating a healthy diet, TCM also emphasizes the importance of proper digestion for healthy skin. In TCM, the digestive system is closely related to the skin, and poor digestion can lead to skin problems such as acne and rosacea. To support healthy digestion and promote healthy skin, TCM recommends eating slowly, chewing food thoroughly, and avoiding overeating or eating too quickly.

When it comes to specific foods and nutrients that are beneficial for promoting healthy skin, TCM emphasizes the importance of incorporating a variety of whole, nutrient-dense foods into the diet. Some of the best foods for promoting healthy skin include:

1. Leafy greens: Leafy greens such as spinach, kale, and collard greens are rich in antioxidants and other nutrients that are beneficial for skin health. They are also a good source of chlorophyll, which can help to promote healthy skin cell growth.

2. Berries: Berries such as blueberries, raspberries, and strawberries are rich in antioxidants, which can help to protect the skin from oxidative stress and promote healthy aging.

3. Nuts and seeds: Nuts and seeds such as almonds, walnuts, and chia seeds are rich in healthy fats, which are essential for maintaining healthy skin. They are also a good source of vitamin E, which is a powerful antioxidant that can help to protect the skin from damage.

4. Fatty fish: Fatty fish such as salmon, sardines, and mackerel are rich in omega-3 fatty acids, which can help to reduce inflammation in the body and promote healthy skin.

5. Bone broth: Bone broth is a nutrient-dense food that is rich in collagen, which is essential for maintaining healthy skin. It is also a good source of minerals such as calcium and magnesium, which are important for overall health.

In addition to these foods,

Foods that nourish and protect the skin

Traditional Chinese Medicine (TCM) emphasizes the importance of internal balance for overall health and well-being, and this includes the health of the skin. According to TCM, the skin reflects the state of the internal organs, and any imbalances or deficiencies can manifest as various skin issues such as acne, eczema, and wrinkles. TCM nutrition focuses on nourishing the body from the inside out to achieve optimal skin health. Here are some foods that are particularly beneficial for the skin.

Green leafy vegetables

Green leafy vegetables such as spinach, kale, and bok choy are packed with nutrients that are essential for healthy skin. They are rich in vitamins A, C, and K, which are necessary for collagen production and repair of damaged skin cells. Additionally, green leafy vegetables contain antioxidants that protect the skin from free radicals and other environmental stressors.

Fruits

Fruits such as berries, oranges, and kiwis are also excellent sources of skin-boosting nutrients. Berries are particularly rich in antioxidants, while oranges are high in vitamin C, which is essential for collagen production. Kiwis, on the other hand, are rich in vitamin E, which helps protect the skin from sun damage.

Bone broth

Bone broth is a nutrient-dense food that is rich in collagen, glucosamine, and other amino acids that support healthy skin. Collagen is the main protein in the skin, and consuming bone broth can help improve skin elasticity and reduce the appearance of wrinkles.

Seafood

Seafood such as salmon, mackerel, and oysters are rich in omega-3 fatty acids, which are essential for healthy skin. Omega-3s can help reduce inflammation and protect the skin from sun damage. Oysters are also a good source of zinc, which is important for collagen production and skin healing.

Tofu

Tofu is a staple in many Asian cuisines and is a good source of protein and isoflavones. Isoflavones are compounds that can help improve skin elasticity and reduce the appearance of wrinkles. Tofu is also rich in antioxidants and can help protect the skin from free radicals.

Nuts and seeds

Nuts and seeds such as almonds, walnuts, and chia seeds are rich in vitamin E, which is important for skin health. Vitamin E is a powerful antioxidant that can help protect the skin from sun damage and reduce inflammation.

Additionally, nuts and seeds contain omega-3s and other healthy fats that support healthy skin.

In addition to incorporating these skin-boosting foods into your diet, there are also some TCM dietary principles that can help improve skin health. One of these principles is to eat a balanced diet that includes a variety of foods. This can help ensure that you are getting all of the nutrients that your skin needs to be healthy. Another principle is to eat foods that are appropriate for your constitution. In TCM, each individual has a unique constitution, and eating foods that are appropriate for your constitution can help improve overall health and skin health.

Chapter Twenty-Four

TCM Nutrition for Strong Bones and Joints

Traditional Chinese Medicine (TCM) has a long history of using food as a way to maintain health and prevent disease. In TCM, strong bones and joints are considered to be the foundation of good health and longevity. There are many dietary strategies that can support strong bones and joints, including the use of certain foods and herbs. Below we will explore TCM nutrition for strong bones and joints, including the key concepts behind this approach, the foods and herbs that are commonly used, and tips for incorporating these strategies into your daily routine.

One of the key concepts behind TCM nutrition for strong bones and joints is the idea of nourishing the Kidneys. In TCM, the Kidneys are considered to be the foundation of good health, and they play a vital role in the growth and development of bones and joints. In order to keep the Kidneys strong and healthy, it is important to eat a balanced diet that is rich in nutrients that support Kidney function.

Some of the key nutrients that support Kidney function and promote strong bones and joints include calcium, magnesium, and vitamin D. Calcium is essential for bone health and is found in many foods, including dairy products, leafy green vegetables, and fortified foods such as orange juice and tofu. Magnesium is also important for bone health and is found in nuts, seeds, and whole grains. Vitamin D is necessary for the absorption of calcium and can be obtained through exposure to sunlight, as well as through dietary sources such as fatty fish and fortified foods.

In addition to these nutrients, there are many foods and herbs that are commonly used in TCM to support strong bones and joints. Some of the most commonly used foods include:

1. Bone Broth: Bone broth is made by simmering bones and connective tissue for an extended period of time. This process releases minerals such as calcium, magnesium, and phosphorus from the bones, making them more easily absorbed by the body. Bone broth is also a good source of collagen, which is important for joint health.

2. Nuts and Seeds: Nuts and seeds are rich in magnesium, which is important for bone health. They also contain healthy fats and protein, which are important for maintaining overall health and well-being.

3. Leafy Green Vegetables: Leafy green vegetables such as kale, spinach, and collard greens are rich in calcium, as well as other important nutrients such as vitamin K and magnesium.

4. Fatty Fish: Fatty fish such as salmon, sardines, and mackerel are a good source of vitamin D, which is necessary for the absorption of calcium.

5. Ginger: Ginger is commonly used in TCM to promote circulation and reduce inflammation. It can be used in cooking or brewed into a tea.

6. Turmeric: Turmeric is a spice that is commonly used in TCM to reduce inflammation. It can be used in cooking or brewed into a tea.

7. Goji Berries: Goji berries are a type of fruit that is commonly used in TCM to promote overall health and well-being. They are rich in antioxidants and are believed to have anti-inflammatory properties.

In addition to these foods, there are also many herbs that are commonly used in TCM to promote strong bones and joints. Some of the most commonly used herbs include:

8. Eucommia: Eucommia is a type of herb that is commonly used in TCM to strengthen the bones and joints. It is believed to promote the production of collagen and other connective tissues.

9. Dipsacus: Dipsacus is a type of herb that is commonly used in TCM to strengthen the bones and promote circulation. It is often used in formulas for treating conditions such as osteoporosis and arthritis.

10. Rehmannia: Re

The role of diet in maintaining bone and joint health

The health of our bones and joints is essential for our mobility and overall well-being. Diet plays an important role in maintaining bone and joint health, and Traditional Chinese Medicine (TCM) offers valuable insights into how we can nourish these parts of our bodies through nutrition.

According to TCM, bone and joint health are closely related to the Kidney and Liver systems. The Kidney system is responsible for our bone health and contains the essence that nourishes our bones, while the Liver system governs the tendons and ligaments that connect our bones and joints.

To support the health of these systems, it is important to consume foods that nourish the Kidney and Liver, as well as those that contain nutrients that are essential for bone and joint health.

One of the key nutrients for bone health is calcium, which is essential for the formation and maintenance of healthy bones. Good dietary sources of calcium include dairy products such as milk, cheese, and yogurt, as well as leafy green vegetables like kale and spinach, and nuts and seeds like almonds and sesame seeds.

Another important nutrient for bone health is vitamin D, which helps the body to absorb calcium. While our bodies can produce vitamin D when our skin is exposed to sunlight, it can be challenging to get enough vitamin D through sunlight alone, especially in the winter months or if you live in a region with limited sun exposure. Good dietary sources of vitamin D include fatty fish like salmon and tuna, egg yolks, and fortified foods like milk and cereals.

In addition to calcium and vitamin D, other nutrients that are important for bone health include magnesium, phosphorus, and vitamin K. Good dietary sources of magnesium include nuts and seeds, legumes, and whole grains. Phosphorus can be found in dairy products, meats, and whole grains, while vitamin K is abundant in leafy green vegetables like spinach and kale.

When it comes to joint health, one of the key nutrients is collagen, which is a type of protein that is found in our bones, tendons, and ligaments. Collagen production declines as we age, which can lead to joint stiffness and pain. Good dietary sources of collagen include bone broth, which is made by simmering animal bones and connective tissues for an extended period of time. Other foods that are rich in collagen include organ meats like liver and heart, as well as gelatin and other collagen supplements.

In addition to these key nutrients, TCM also recommends consuming foods that nourish the Kidney and Liver systems, as these systems are closely related to bone and joint health. Foods that are good for the Kidney system include black beans, kidney beans, and black sesame seeds, while foods that are good for the Liver system include bitter greens like dandelion greens and arugula, as well as sour foods like vinegar and citrus fruits.

It is also important to pay attention to cooking methods when preparing foods for bone and joint health. TCM recommends cooking methods that are gentle and do not overly dry out or damage the food. For example, steaming, boiling, and stewing are good cooking methods, while frying and grilling should be avoided or minimized.

Incorporating TCM nutrition principles into your diet can help to support the health of your bones and joints, as well as your overall well-being. By consuming foods that are rich in key nutrients like calcium, vitamin D, and collagen, as well as those that nourish the Kidney and Liver systems, you can help to promote strong bones and healthy joints for years to come.

Foods that support bone and joint strength

Foods play a vital role in maintaining bone and joint health. According to Traditional Chinese Medicine (TCM), our diet can impact the health of our bones and joints. TCM emphasizes the importance of a balanced diet that includes various nutrient-rich foods to support optimal bone and joint health. Below we will explore some of the foods that can support bone and joint strength from a TCM perspective.

1. Leafy greens: Leafy greens are a great source of calcium, which is an essential mineral for bone health. Examples of leafy greens include kale, spinach, bok choy, and collard greens. In TCM, leafy greens are believed to nourish the Liver and promote blood circulation, which can support joint health.

2. Bone broth: Bone broth is a nutrient-rich food that is made by simmering animal bones and connective tissue. It is a rich source of collagen, which is a protein that plays a vital role in joint health. Collagen provides the building blocks for bones, tendons, and ligaments, and consuming bone broth can help support the health of these structures.

3. Fish: Fish is a rich source of omega-3 fatty acids, which have been shown to support joint health by reducing inflammation. Examples of fish that are high in omega-3s include salmon, sardines, and mackerel. In TCM, fish is believed to nourish the Kidneys, which are the organs responsible for bone health.

4. Nuts and seeds: Nuts and seeds are a great source of minerals, including calcium, magnesium, and zinc, which are all essential for bone health. Examples of nuts and seeds that are particularly beneficial for bone health include almonds, sesame seeds, and pumpkin seeds. In TCM, nuts and seeds are believed to support the Kidneys, which can help promote strong bones.

5. Berries: Berries are a great source of antioxidants, which can help protect the joints from damage caused by free radicals. Examples of berries that are particularly beneficial for joint health include blueberries, raspberries, and blackberries. In TCM, berries are believed to nourish the Liver, which can help promote healthy joints.

6. Garlic: Garlic is a great source of sulfur, which is an essential mineral for joint health. Sulfur is needed to produce collagen, which is essential for healthy joints. In TCM, garlic is believed to nourish the Lungs, which can help promote healthy bones and joints.

7. Turmeric: Turmeric is a spice that has been shown to have anti-inflammatory properties, which can help support joint health. In TCM, turmeric is believed to promote blood circulation and reduce inflammation, which can help support healthy bones and joints.

Chapter Twenty-Five

TCM Nutrition for Heart Health

Traditional Chinese Medicine (TCM) is a holistic approach to healthcare that includes the use of natural remedies, including dietary changes, to support overall health and wellbeing. One area where TCM nutrition can be particularly beneficial is in supporting heart health.

In TCM, the heart is seen as the organ that controls the flow of blood and the energy, or qi, throughout the body. When the heart is healthy, the blood and qi flow smoothly, supporting overall health and vitality. However, when the heart is imbalanced, the body may experience a range of symptoms, including palpitations, shortness of breath, and fatigue.

To support heart health in TCM, there are several dietary recommendations that can be followed. One key principle is to consume a diet that is low in saturated fat and high in fiber. This can help to reduce inflammation in the body, which can be a risk factor for heart disease. Additionally, consuming a diet rich in antioxidants can help to protect the heart and blood vessels from damage caused by free radicals.

Some specific foods that are recommended for heart health in TCM include:

1. Whole grains: Whole grains, such as brown rice and oats, are high in fiber and can help to lower cholesterol levels, reducing the risk of heart disease.

2. Leafy green vegetables: Leafy green vegetables, such as kale and spinach, are rich in antioxidants and other nutrients that support heart health.

3. Berries: Berries, such as blueberries and raspberries, are high in antioxidants and can help to protect the heart and blood vessels from damage caused by free radicals.

4. Legumes: Legumes, such as lentils and chickpeas, are high in fiber and protein and can help to reduce cholesterol levels and support overall heart health.

5. Nuts and seeds: Nuts and seeds, such as almonds and chia seeds, are rich in healthy fats and other nutrients that support heart health.

In addition to incorporating these foods into the diet, there are also some cooking techniques that are recommended in TCM to support heart health. One key principle is to avoid deep-frying or cooking foods at high temperatures, as this can create harmful compounds that can damage the heart and blood vessels. Instead, cooking methods such as steaming, boiling, and stir-frying are recommended.

Finally, in TCM, it is also important to consider the emotional aspect of heart health. The heart is seen as the center of emotions, and emotional stress can have a significant impact on heart health. Therefore, it is recommended to cultivate a sense of calm and relaxation in daily life through practices such as meditation, deep breathing, and gentle exercise such as tai chi or yoga.

The importance of heart health in TCM

Traditional Chinese Medicine (TCM) places great emphasis on the health of the heart, recognizing it as the center of vitality and energy in the body. According to TCM, the heart governs blood circulation and is responsible for the proper functioning of all the organs and systems in the body. A healthy heart is essential for maintaining optimal health and preventing disease. Below we will explore the importance of heart health in TCM and how nutrition plays a crucial role in maintaining a healthy heart.

In TCM, the heart is considered one of the five vital organs, along with the liver, spleen, lungs, and kidneys. Each of these organs is connected to specific emotions, and the heart is associated with joy and happiness. When the heart is healthy, it is said to be in a state of balance, and a person experiences a sense of calmness, contentment, and emotional stability. However, when the heart is imbalanced, it can lead to a range of physical and emotional symptoms.

According to TCM, there are several factors that can lead to heart imbalances, including poor diet, stress, and emotional imbalances. A poor diet, in particular, can lead to the accumulation of toxins in the body, which can impair heart function and lead to a range of cardiovascular diseases. Therefore, it is essential to follow a healthy diet that supports heart health.

One of the primary principles of TCM nutrition is the importance of balance. In TCM, it is believed that the body is in a state of balance when it is in harmony with nature. This means that the body is nourished with a variety of whole foods that are in season and grown locally. Eating a balanced diet that includes a variety of whole foods, such as fruits, vegetables, whole grains, and lean proteins, is essential for maintaining a healthy heart.

Certain foods and herbs are also believed to be beneficial for heart health in TCM. For example, foods that are rich in antioxidants, such as blueberries, goji berries, and dark leafy greens, are believed to help protect the heart from oxidative stress and inflammation. Other heart-healthy foods include oily fish, nuts and seeds, and whole grains.

In addition to diet, lifestyle factors also play a crucial role in maintaining heart health in TCM. Regular exercise, stress management techniques, and getting enough rest are all important for maintaining a healthy heart. In

TCM, stress is believed to be a significant contributor to heart imbalances, so it is essential to find ways to manage stress effectively, such as through meditation, yoga, or deep breathing exercises.

Herbs are also used in TCM to support heart health. For example, hawthorn berry is believed to strengthen the heart muscle, improve circulation, and reduce high blood pressure. Other herbs that are used for heart health in TCM include red sage root, ginseng, and dan shen.

Foods that support cardiovascular health

Traditional Chinese Medicine (TCM) has long recognized the importance of maintaining good heart health. According to TCM, the heart is the emperor of the body and is responsible for circulating blood and controlling emotions. Therefore, it is essential to take care of the heart to maintain overall well-being. Nutrition plays a crucial role in supporting heart health in TCM. Below we will explore some foods that are believed to be beneficial for cardiovascular health.

Oats

Oats are a heart-healthy food that is commonly used in TCM. They are rich in fiber, which can help lower cholesterol levels in the blood. Oats are also an excellent source of magnesium, a mineral that plays a vital role in maintaining a healthy heart rhythm. In TCM, oats are considered a nourishing food for the heart and are often used in tonics and herbal formulas.

Garlic

Garlic is a pungent herb that has been used for centuries for its medicinal properties. It contains a compound called allicin, which has been shown to have anti-inflammatory and antiplatelet effects, both of which can benefit heart health. Garlic has also been shown to help lower blood pressure, which is a risk factor for heart disease.

Salmon

Salmon is a fatty fish that is rich in omega-3 fatty acids, which are essential for heart health. Omega-3 fatty acids have been shown to help lower triglycerides, reduce inflammation, and decrease the risk of arrhythmias. In TCM, salmon is considered a cooling food that can help reduce inflammation in the body.

Berries

Berries are an excellent source of antioxidants, which can help protect the heart from oxidative stress. They are also rich in fiber, which can help lower cholesterol levels in the blood. In TCM, berries are considered a nourishing food that can help tonify the blood.

Green Tea

Green tea is a popular beverage in TCM and is known for its antioxidant properties. It contains catechins, a type of antioxidant that has been shown to have cardio-protective effects. Green tea has also been shown to help lower blood pressure and improve cholesterol levels in the blood.

Turmeric

Turmeric is a spice that is commonly used in TCM for its anti-inflammatory properties. It contains a compound called curcumin, which has been shown to have cardioprotective effects. Curcumin has been shown to help lower blood pressure, reduce inflammation, and improve cholesterol levels in the blood.

Nuts

Nuts are a heart-healthy food that is rich in monounsaturated and polyunsaturated fats, which can help improve cholesterol levels in the blood. They are also a good source of fiber, which can help lower the risk of heart disease. In TCM, nuts are considered a nourishing food that can help strengthen the kidneys, which are closely linked to heart health.

Sweet Potatoes

Sweet potatoes are a heart-healthy food that is rich in fiber, vitamins, and minerals. They are also a good source of antioxidants, which can help protect the heart from oxidative stress. In TCM, sweet potatoes are considered a nourishing food that can help tonify the spleen and stomach, which are essential for proper digestion and absorption of nutrients.

Spinach

Spinach is a leafy green vegetable that is rich in vitamins, minerals, and antioxidants. It is also a good source of nitrates, which can help improve blood flow and lower blood pressure. In TCM, spinach is considered a cooling food that can help clear heat from the body.

Dark Chocolate

Dark chocolate is a delicious treat that is also good for the heart. It contains flavonoids, a type of antioxidant that

Chapter Twenty-Six

TCM Nutrition for Better Sleep

TCM, or Traditional Chinese Medicine, has a holistic approach to health and wellness, recognizing that every aspect of our being is interconnected. This includes the relationship between our nutrition and sleep. In TCM, sleep is considered essential for good health, as it allows the body to rest, recover and restore itself. Conversely, poor sleep quality or lack of sleep can lead to a host of physical and mental health issues.

Fortunately, TCM offers many dietary recommendations and strategies to improve sleep quality and duration. Here are some key TCM nutrition tips for better sleep:

1. Eat Foods that Nourish the Yin: In TCM, sleep is considered a yin activity, which means that it is associated with quiet, coolness, and relaxation. Eating foods that nourish the yin can help support better sleep. These foods include leafy greens, mushrooms, seaweed, beans, tofu, and fish.

2. Avoid Foods that Create Excess Heat: In contrast to yin foods, yang foods are associated with activity, heat, and stimulation. Eating too many yang foods can disrupt the balance of yin and yang in the body, making it harder to fall and stay asleep. Yang foods include spicy or greasy foods, caffeine, alcohol, and meat.

3. Incorporate Foods with Sleep-Promoting Nutrients: Certain nutrients can help promote sleep, such as magnesium, tryptophan, and melatonin.

Foods that contain these nutrients include leafy greens, almonds, oats, bananas, and tart cherry juice.

4. Eat Regularly and Avoid Late-Night Meals: In TCM, digestion is a yang activity, so eating late at night can create excess yang energy, making it harder to fall asleep. Aim to eat regular meals throughout the day and avoid eating large meals or snacks close to bedtime.

5. Mindful Eating: In addition to choosing the right foods, TCM also emphasizes the importance of mindful eating. This means taking the time to savor and appreciate your food, eating in a relaxed and peaceful environment, and avoiding distractions such as screens or stressful conversations.

6. Herbal Supplements: In addition to food, TCM also incorporates herbal supplements to support better sleep. These may include herbs such as valerian root, passionflower, and chamomile, which have calming and relaxing properties.

Incorporating TCM nutrition tips into your daily routine can help support better sleep and overall health. It is important to remember that every person is unique, and what works for one person may not work for another. If you are struggling with sleep issues, it may be helpful to consult with a TCM practitioner who can offer personalized recommendations and support.

The connection between diet and sleep quality

The importance of good sleep cannot be overemphasized. Adequate sleep is essential for physical and mental health, including better cognitive function, a stronger immune system, and lower risk of chronic diseases. Unfortunately, sleep disorders are becoming more common, and many people suffer from poor sleep quality. While there are various factors that can impact sleep, including stress, environment, and lifestyle, diet also plays a significant role in regulating sleep quality.

Traditional Chinese Medicine (TCM) recognizes that nutrition plays a vital role in sleep quality. According to TCM, sleep disorders are often caused by imbalances in the body's energy, or Qi. Therefore, maintaining a balanced diet that supports the flow of Qi throughout the body is essential for improving sleep quality.

One key aspect of TCM nutrition for better sleep is the timing and quantity of food intake. It is generally recommended to avoid heavy meals before bedtime as they can interfere with digestion and disrupt sleep. Instead, TCM suggests eating smaller, lighter meals earlier in the evening, preferably at least two hours before bedtime. This allows the body to digest food properly and prevent discomfort that could keep you up at night.

Another essential aspect of TCM nutrition for better sleep is the choice of foods. In TCM, foods are categorized according to their energetic properties, including their effect on Qi flow. For example, foods that are considered warming, such as ginger and cinnamon, promote circulation and help disperse cold, which can negatively affect sleep. Other foods, such as fruits and leafy greens, are considered cooling and help calm the body.

In addition, TCM emphasizes the importance of consuming foods that nourish the heart and calm the mind. The heart in TCM is responsible for regulating sleep, and consuming foods that support its function can improve sleep quality. Foods such as walnuts, almonds, and flaxseeds are rich in omega-3 fatty acids, which support heart health and can help reduce anxiety and depression, leading to better sleep.

TCM also recommends consuming foods that support the liver, which plays a crucial role in maintaining the body's energy balance. When the liver is overworked, it can lead to imbalances in Qi flow and disrupt sleep.

Foods that support liver function include leafy greens, beets, carrots, and citrus fruits, which are rich in antioxidants and can help reduce inflammation and protect the liver.

Lastly, TCM also recommends consuming foods that promote relaxation and calmness. Chamomile tea, for example, is well known for its calming effects and is a popular natural remedy for promoting sleep. Other foods that can help promote relaxation include lavender, passionflower, and valerian root.

Foods that promote restful sleep

Foods and nutrients have been found to play a crucial role in regulating sleep. In Traditional Chinese Medicine (TCM), certain foods and herbs are believed to promote restful sleep by nourishing the body and mind, calming the spirit, and harmonizing the Qi. Below we will discuss some of the best foods and nutrients for promoting restful sleep according to TCM.

Firstly, TCM practitioners believe that the spleen and stomach are the organs responsible for transforming food into Qi and blood, which are essential for a healthy body and mind. Therefore, eating foods that support spleen and stomach function is believed to help promote restful sleep. These foods include whole grains, sweet potatoes, carrots, pumpkins, and other root vegetables. They are high in complex carbohydrates, which provide a steady source of energy and prevent blood sugar spikes and crashes that can interfere with sleep.

Another essential nutrient for sleep is magnesium, which plays a crucial role in regulating the body's stress response and promoting relaxation. Magnesium-rich foods include leafy green vegetables such as spinach and kale, nuts and seeds such as almonds and pumpkin seeds, and legumes such as lentils and black beans. Eating these foods regularly can help promote restful sleep.

In TCM, certain herbs are also believed to be beneficial for promoting restful sleep. For example, chamomile tea has been used for centuries as a natural sleep aid. It contains compounds that have a calming effect on the nervous system and promote relaxation. Other herbs commonly used in TCM for promoting restful sleep include valerian root, passionflower, and skullcap.

In addition to specific foods and herbs, TCM practitioners also emphasize the importance of eating a balanced and varied diet to promote overall health and wellbeing. Eating a diet rich in fresh fruits and vegetables, whole grains, lean protein sources, and healthy fats is believed to support overall health and contribute to restful sleep.

Finally, TCM practitioners also recommend avoiding certain foods and lifestyle habits that can interfere with sleep. For example, caffeine, alcohol, and nicotine are all stimulants that can disrupt sleep patterns. Eating heavy or spicy meals before bedtime can also interfere with sleep, as can engaging in stimulating activities such as using electronic devices or watching television in the hours leading up to bedtime.

Chapter Twenty-Seven

TCM Nutrition for Stress Management

TCM (Traditional Chinese Medicine) is a holistic approach to health and wellness that has been practiced for over 2,500 years. One of the core principles of TCM is the idea that emotional and mental health are deeply connected to physical health. This is especially true when it comes to stress, which is a common issue in modern society. Stress can have a significant impact on overall health, and if not managed properly, it can lead to a variety of health problems. TCM offers a range of nutritional strategies to support stress management and promote overall wellness.

The Role of Diet in Stress Management in TCM

In TCM, the idea of nourishing the body to achieve balance and harmony is emphasized. This means that the foods you eat play a vital role in managing stress. A healthy diet is essential for supporting the body's natural healing mechanisms, promoting overall wellness, and managing stress.

According to TCM, stress can disrupt the flow of Qi (energy) in the body, leading to a variety of physical and emotional symptoms. When the body is stressed, the Qi can become stagnant or blocked, leading to imbalances and health problems. TCM nutrition focuses on promoting the flow of Qi and restoring balance to the body.

Foods that Promote Stress Management in TCM

1. Whole grains: Whole grains such as brown rice, quinoa, and millet are rich in nutrients and fiber, which can help support digestive health and promote a sense of fullness. In TCM, whole grains are considered to be nourishing and grounding, helping to calm the mind and reduce stress.

2. Leafy Greens: Leafy greens such as spinach, kale, and collard greens are rich in nutrients and antioxidants, which can help support overall health and reduce inflammation in the body. In TCM, leafy greens are considered to be cooling and cleansing, helping to balance the body and promote relaxation.

3. Root vegetables: Root vegetables such as sweet potatoes, carrots, and beets are rich in nutrients and fiber, which can help support digestive health and promote a sense of fullness. In TCM, root vegetables are considered to be nourishing and grounding, helping to calm the mind and reduce stress.

4. Herbal teas: Herbal teas such as chamomile, lavender, and lemon balm are known for their calming properties and can help promote relaxation and reduce stress. In TCM, these teas are considered to be cooling and calming, helping to balance the body and promote a sense of peace.

5. Nuts and seeds: Nuts and seeds such as almonds, walnuts, and pumpkin seeds are rich in healthy fats, protein, and fiber, which can help support overall health and reduce inflammation in the body. In TCM, nuts and seeds are considered to be nourishing and grounding, helping to calm the mind and reduce stress.

6. Fermented foods: Fermented foods such as sauerkraut, kimchi, and kefir are rich in beneficial bacteria, which can help support digestive health and promote overall wellness. In TCM, fermented foods are considered to be warming and nourishing, helping to balance the body and promote relaxation.

TCM Nutrition Strategies for Managing Stress

In addition to eating a balanced diet, there are several other TCM nutrition strategies that can help manage stress and promote overall wellness.

7. Eating mindfully: Eating mindfully means paying attention to the present moment, savoring each bite, and taking the time to enjoy your food. This can help reduce stress and promote a sense of calm and relaxation.

8. Eating regular meals: Eating regular meals can help regulate blood sugar levels and prevent energy dips, which can contribute to stress and anxiety.

9. Drinking plenty of water: Staying hydrated is essential for maintaining optimal health and managing stress

The impact of stress on health in TCM

Traditional Chinese Medicine (TCM) recognizes that stress can negatively impact overall health and well-being. In TCM theory, stress can lead to an imbalance in the body's vital energy, or qi, which can manifest as physical or emotional symptoms. Therefore, managing stress is an important aspect of maintaining good health in TCM.

Stress can affect the body in several ways. For example, it can lead to hormonal imbalances, which can cause changes in appetite, mood, and energy levels. Chronic stress can also increase inflammation and oxidative stress, which are associated with numerous health problems, including heart disease, diabetes, and cancer.

In TCM, stress is often associated with the liver system. The liver is responsible for regulating the flow of qi and blood throughout the body, and stress can cause the liver to become stagnant or congested. This can lead to symptoms such as irritability, anger, and headaches.

To support the liver and manage stress in TCM, it is important to follow a balanced and nourishing diet. Some foods and dietary practices that can help manage stress include:

1. Eat a variety of nutrient-dense foods: Eating a diverse range of nutrient-rich foods can help ensure that the body has the vitamins and minerals it needs to function properly. This includes plenty of fresh fruits and vegetables, whole grains, lean protein, and healthy fats.

2. Avoid processed and refined foods: Processed and refined foods, such as sugary snacks, white bread, and fast food, can cause blood sugar spikes and crashes, which can contribute to stress and fatigue.

3. Incorporate stress-reducing foods: Certain foods are known to have stress-reducing properties, such as chamomile tea, dark chocolate, and omega-3-rich fatty fish like salmon.

4. Practice mindful eating: Eating mindfully, or paying attention to the experience of eating without distraction, can help reduce stress and improve digestion. This can be achieved by eating slowly, savoring the flavors and textures of food, and avoiding multitasking while eating.

5. Avoid overeating: Overeating can lead to discomfort and digestive issues, which can contribute to stress and anxiety.

6. Cook meals at home: Cooking meals at home with fresh, whole ingredients can help ensure that the body receives the nutrients it needs and can be a relaxing and enjoyable activity.

7. Limit caffeine and alcohol: Caffeine and alcohol can disrupt sleep and contribute to feelings of anxiety and stress. Limiting or avoiding these substances can help improve sleep and reduce stress.

In addition to these dietary practices, other TCM practices can also help manage stress. These include acupuncture, herbal remedies, meditation, and tai chi. These practices can help balance the flow of qi and promote relaxation and a sense of calm.

Foods that help alleviate stress

In Traditional Chinese Medicine (TCM), food is considered not only as a source of nutrition but also as a form of medicine that can help prevent and treat various health conditions. One of the most common health issues that TCM addresses is stress. Stress can lead to a wide range of health problems, such as anxiety, depression, insomnia, and digestive issues. In TCM, the goal is to achieve a balance of yin and yang, and the foods we eat can either support or disrupt that balance. Here are some foods that can help alleviate stress and promote a sense of calmness in the body.

Leafy Greens

Leafy greens, such as spinach, kale, and collard greens, are rich in magnesium. Magnesium is an essential mineral that plays a crucial role in reducing stress and anxiety by regulating the production of cortisol, a stress hormone. Studies have shown that magnesium deficiency is linked to an increased risk of anxiety and depression. Including leafy greens in your diet can help ensure that you're getting enough magnesium.

Nuts and Seeds

Nuts and seeds, such as almonds, walnuts, and pumpkin seeds, are also rich in magnesium. They are also a good source of protein and healthy fats, which can help stabilize blood sugar levels and prevent mood swings. Additionally, they contain amino acids that help promote the production of serotonin, a neurotransmitter that regulates mood and promotes feelings of happiness.

Fatty Fish

Fatty fish, such as salmon, tuna, and sardines, are high in omega-3 fatty acids, which have been shown to reduce inflammation and promote brain health. Studies have also found that omega-3 fatty acids can help alleviate symptoms of anxiety and depression.

Turmeric

Turmeric is a spice that has been used in Ayurvedic and TCM medicine for centuries. It contains curcumin, a compound that has anti-inflammatory and antioxidant properties. Studies have shown that curcumin can help reduce symptoms of depression and anxiety.

Chamomile Tea

Chamomile tea is a popular herbal tea that is known for its calming effects. It contains apigenin, a flavonoid that binds to specific receptors in the brain, promoting relaxation and reducing anxiety.

Fermented Foods

Fermented foods, such as kimchi, sauerkraut, and kefir, contain probiotics that help promote gut health. Studies have found that the gut-brain axis plays a crucial role in regulating mood and stress levels. Fermented foods can help restore balance to the gut microbiome, promoting overall health and well-being.

Dark Chocolate

Dark chocolate is a rich source of antioxidants and contains compounds that have been shown to reduce stress and anxiety. It also contains magnesium, which can help regulate cortisol levels.

Incorporating these foods into your diet can help promote a sense of calmness and reduce stress levels. However, it's important to remember that a healthy diet is just one aspect of stress management. Other factors, such as exercise, sleep, and social support, also play a crucial role in reducing stress levels. By taking a holistic approach to stress management, you can help promote overall health and well-being.

Chapter Twenty-Eight

TCM Nutrition for Immune System Support

Traditional Chinese Medicine (TCM) has a long history of using food as a way to support and strengthen the immune system. In TCM, it is believed that maintaining a balanced diet is one of the most effective ways to maintain good health and prevent illness. There are several key principles of TCM nutrition that can help boost the immune system and promote overall health and wellness.

The first principle of TCM nutrition is to consume a balanced diet that includes a variety of different foods. This means including foods from all of the different food groups, such as whole grains, vegetables, fruits, lean proteins, and healthy fats. It is also important to eat foods that are in season and locally sourced whenever possible, as this can help support the body's natural rhythms and promote optimal health.

Another important principle of TCM nutrition is to focus on consuming whole, nutrient-dense foods. This means avoiding highly processed foods that are high in sugar, salt, and unhealthy fats, as these can lead to inflammation and weaken the immune system. Instead, choose foods that are high in vitamins, minerals, and antioxidants, such as leafy greens, berries, nuts and seeds, and lean proteins like fish and chicken.

In TCM, there are several specific foods and herbs that are known to support immune system function. One of the most popular of these is astragalus root, which is believed to help boost the immune system and reduce inflammation. Other immune-boosting foods and herbs include medicinal mushrooms like shiitake and reishi, garlic, ginger, and green tea.

One important aspect of TCM nutrition for immune system support is to pay attention to food energetics. In TCM, each food is believed to have its own unique energetic properties that can affect the body in different ways. For example, some foods are believed to be warming, while others are cooling. By eating a variety of different foods that have different energetic properties, you can help balance the body and support optimal health.

TCM also emphasizes the importance of good digestion for immune system function. When the digestive system is working properly, the body is better able to absorb the nutrients it needs to support immune system function. Eating slowly, chewing thoroughly, and consuming foods that are easy to digest can all help support good digestive health.

In addition to focusing on a balanced and nutrient-dense diet, there are several other TCM practices that can help support immune system function. These include getting plenty of restful sleep, managing stress levels, and engaging in regular physical activity. When the body is well-rested, relaxed, and active, it is better equipped to fight off infections and maintain optimal health.

The importance of a strong immune system in TCM

Traditional Chinese Medicine (TCM) has been promoting the importance of a strong immune system for thousands of years. The immune system is crucial in TCM because it is considered to be the body's primary line of defense against illness and disease. In TCM, the immune system is closely linked with the body's energy or "Qi," and a deficiency in Qi can result in a weakened immune system. Therefore, it is essential to maintain a healthy immune system through a balanced diet and lifestyle, as well as incorporating TCM practices.

One of the primary focuses of TCM nutrition for immune system support is to nourish the body and provide it with the nutrients it needs to function properly. This means incorporating a variety of whole foods, including fruits, vegetables, whole grains, and lean protein sources into the diet. It is also recommended to eat a variety of colors, as different colors in food provide different nutrients and antioxidants that support the immune system.

In TCM, certain foods are believed to have specific properties that can support the immune system. For example, mushrooms, including shiitake, maitake, and reishi, are known for their immune-boosting properties. They contain polysaccharides, which stimulate the immune system and enhance its ability to fight off infections and diseases. Additionally, garlic and onions are known for their antiviral and antibacterial properties and can help the body fight off infections. Other foods that are believed to support the immune system include ginger, turmeric, green tea, and goji berries.

In addition to incorporating immune-boosting foods into the diet, TCM also recommends a balanced lifestyle to support the immune system. This includes getting enough rest, managing stress, and engaging in regular physical activity. Adequate sleep is essential for the immune system, as it allows the body to repair and regenerate. Stress management is also crucial because stress can weaken the immune system over time. Engaging in regular physical activity helps to strengthen the immune system, as exercise can help increase the circulation of immune cells throughout the body.

TCM also recommends avoiding certain foods that can weaken the immune system. These include processed foods, refined sugar, and excessive alcohol consumption. These foods can cause inflammation in the body, which can impair the immune system's ability to function properly. It is also important to limit the consumption of cold and raw foods, as these can weaken the digestive system, which is closely linked to the immune system in TCM.

Finally, TCM practices such as acupuncture and herbal medicine can also be used to support the immune system. Acupuncture has been shown to increase the circulation of immune cells in the body, while herbal medicine can provide specific nutrients and compounds that support the immune system. For example, astragalus root is commonly used in TCM as an immune-boosting herb.

Foods that boost immunity

Traditional Chinese Medicine (TCM) places great emphasis on the importance of a strong immune system. In TCM, the immune system is closely linked with the concept of Wei Qi, which is the body's protective energy. According to TCM principles, the strength of Wei Qi determines our ability to resist disease and maintain good health. Proper nutrition plays a crucial role in supporting the immune system, and TCM offers a variety of foods that can boost immunity and enhance overall health.

One of the key principles of TCM nutrition is the importance of consuming a balanced diet that includes a variety of nutrient-dense foods. TCM practitioners believe that a balanced diet can help to support the body's natural healing abilities, including the immune system. They recommend incorporating a variety of foods that nourish the body and provide it with the energy it needs to stay healthy.

In TCM, foods are classified according to their energetic properties, which are believed to have a direct impact on the body. For example, some foods are considered to be warming and are believed to help stimulate circulation and promote the movement of Qi (energy) in the body. Other foods are considered to be cooling and are believed to help soothe inflammation and reduce heat in the body. By choosing foods that are appropriate for your individual constitution and health needs, you can help to support your immune system and promote overall wellness.

One of the best ways to boost immunity through nutrition is by consuming a variety of colorful fruits and vegetables. These foods are packed with vitamins, minerals, and antioxidants that can help to support the immune system and protect the body against disease. Some particularly beneficial foods include:

1. Mushrooms: Various types of mushrooms have been used in TCM for centuries to support immune function. Shiitake, maitake, and reishi mushrooms, in particular, contain beta-glucans, which are believed to enhance the immune response by activating certain immune cells.

2. Berries: Berries are a rich source of antioxidants, which can help to protect the body against damage from free radicals. Blueberries, blackberries, and raspberries are particularly high in anthocyanins, which have been shown to boost immunity and reduce inflammation.

3. Citrus fruits: Citrus fruits like oranges, lemons, and grapefruits are rich in vitamin C, which is essential for immune function. Vitamin C helps to stimulate the production of white blood cells, which play a crucial role in fighting off infections.

4. Garlic: Garlic has long been used in TCM to support immune function. It contains a compound called allicin, which has been shown to have antibacterial and antiviral properties.

5. Ginger: Ginger is another TCM staple that has been used for centuries to support immune function. It contains gingerols and shogaols, which are believed to have anti-inflammatory and immune-boosting properties.

In addition to incorporating immune-boosting foods into your diet, TCM practitioners also recommend practicing mindful eating habits. This includes chewing food thoroughly, eating slowly, and avoiding overeating or consuming large meals late at night. They also recommend avoiding foods that are overly processed, high in sugar, or difficult to digest, as these can all place a burden on the immune system and contribute to inflammation.

Finally, TCM practitioners recommend focusing on overall lifestyle habits that support the immune system. This includes getting enough sleep, managing stress, staying physically active, and avoiding exposure to toxins and environmental pollutants.

Chapter Twenty-Nine

TCM Nutrition for Brain Health and Cognitive Function

TCM (Traditional Chinese Medicine) has a long history of utilizing nutrition as a key component of maintaining optimal health. In TCM, the brain and the body are interconnected, and proper nutrition can play a significant role in cognitive function and overall brain health. Below we will explore the various TCM principles and dietary recommendations that can help promote better brain health and cognitive function.

The Importance of Brain Health in TCM

In TCM, the brain is considered to be the "Sea of Marrow," responsible for our mental activities, emotions, and senses. The concept of "Qi," which translates to "vital energy," is also central to TCM. It is believed that the Qi flows throughout the body, and any blockages or imbalances can lead to various health issues, including those related to brain health and cognitive function.

TCM practitioners often use acupuncture, herbal remedies, and dietary recommendations to address imbalances in the body's Qi and promote overall health. A balanced diet is crucial for maintaining Qi flow and good brain health, and certain foods are believed to have a positive impact on cognitive function.

Foods that Promote Brain Health and Cognitive Function

Nuts and Seeds

Nuts and seeds are a great source of healthy fats, vitamins, and minerals that are essential for brain health. For example, walnuts are rich in omega-3 fatty acids, which have been linked to improved brain function and decreased cognitive decline. Almonds are another great option, as they are high in vitamin E, which can help improve memory and cognitive function.

Dark Leafy Greens

Dark leafy greens, such as spinach and kale, are rich in antioxidants and vitamins that are essential for brain health. These vegetables are high in vitamin K, which has been linked to improved cognitive function and a reduced risk of Alzheimer's disease.

Berries

Berries, such as blueberries and strawberries, are packed with antioxidants and other compounds that can help protect the brain from damage caused by free radicals. They are also high in flavonoids, which have been linked to improved memory and cognitive function.

Fish

Fish, such as salmon and tuna, are high in omega-3 fatty acids, which have been linked to improved brain function and a reduced risk of cognitive decline. These fatty acids can also help reduce inflammation in the brain and improve mood.

Whole Grains

Whole grains, such as brown rice and quinoa, are rich in fiber, vitamins, and minerals that are essential for brain health. These grains are high in B vitamins, which have been linked to improved cognitive function and a reduced risk of dementia.

TCM Principles for Brain Health

In addition to incorporating brain-boosting foods into your diet, TCM principles can also be applied to promote brain health and cognitive function. Here are some TCM recommendations for maintaining optimal brain health:

Balance Yin and Yang

In TCM, Yin and Yang are considered to be opposing forces that need to be balanced for optimal health. An excess of Yang energy can lead to inflammation and oxidative stress in the brain, while an excess of Yin energy can lead to sluggishness and poor brain function. Balancing these energies through a proper diet and lifestyle can help promote better brain health.

Address Deficiencies

TCM practitioners often look for deficiencies in the body that may be contributing to poor brain function. For example, a deficiency in the Qi or blood can lead to poor brain function and cognitive decline. Addressing these deficiencies through diet and herbal remedies can help improve brain health.

Reduce Stress

Stress can be a significant contributor to poor brain function and cognitive decline. TCM recommends reducing stress through practices such as meditation, acupuncture, and herbal remedies. A balanced diet can also help reduce stress and

The connection between diet and brain health

The food we eat has a significant impact on our overall health, including our brain health and cognitive function. In Traditional Chinese Medicine (TCM), the connection between diet and brain health has been recognized for thousands of years. TCM practitioners believe that the food we eat can influence our brain function, mood, and memory. Below we will explore the connection between diet and brain health and discuss some of the TCM principles that guide us in making healthy food choices for our brains.

The human brain is the most complex organ in the body, and it requires a constant supply of energy and nutrients to function properly. A diet that is high in processed foods, sugar, and unhealthy fats can contribute to chronic inflammation, which can impair cognitive function and increase the risk of developing conditions such as Alzheimer's disease and other forms of dementia. Conversely, a diet that is rich in whole foods, healthy fats, and antioxidants can help to protect the brain from damage and promote optimal cognitive function.

One of the key principles of TCM nutrition is that food should be consumed in a way that balances the body's energy, or qi. According to TCM, the brain is nourished by the kidney and liver systems, which are responsible for filtering and detoxifying the blood. Therefore, foods that support these systems can help to promote optimal brain health. Some of the foods that are recommended for kidney and liver health in TCM include:

1. Leafy greens: Leafy greens such as kale, spinach, and collard greens are rich in vitamins and minerals that support kidney and liver function. They are also high in antioxidants, which help to protect the brain from damage caused by free radicals.

2. Fish: Cold-water fatty fish such as salmon, sardines, and mackerel are high in omega-3 fatty acids, which have been shown to improve cognitive function and protect against age-related cognitive decline.

3. Nuts and seeds: Nuts and seeds such as almonds, walnuts, and chia seeds are high in healthy fats and antioxidants, which can help to protect the brain from inflammation and oxidative stress.

4. Berries: Berries such as blueberries, blackberries, and strawberries are high in antioxidants and have been shown to improve cognitive function and protect against age-related cognitive decline.

5. Whole grains: Whole grains such as brown rice, quinoa, and oats are rich in fiber and B vitamins, which support healthy brain function and help to regulate mood.

Another key principle of TCM nutrition is that food should be consumed in a way that supports the body's natural rhythms. TCM practitioners believe that our bodies have an internal clock that governs our sleep-wake cycles, digestion, and other bodily functions. Eating at regular intervals and avoiding heavy meals before bedtime can help to regulate these rhythms and promote optimal brain function.

TCM also recognizes the importance of balancing the five elements in our diets. According to TCM, the five elements (wood, fire, earth, metal, and water) correspond to different organs and bodily functions. For example, the element of fire is associated with the heart, while the element of water is associated with the kidneys. Eating a variety of foods from each of the five elements can help to balance the body's energy and promote optimal brain health.

In addition to these principles, there are also specific foods and herbs that are commonly used in TCM to promote brain health and cognitive function. Some of these include:

6. Gingko biloba: Gingko biloba is an herb that has been shown to improve cognitive function and memory in people with Alzheimer's disease and other forms of dementia.

7. Gotu kola: Gotu kola is an herb that has been traditionally used in TCM to improve memory and cognitive function.

8. Ginseng: Gins

Foods that support cognitive function

Foods have a significant impact on our physical and mental health, including our cognitive function. In Traditional Chinese Medicine (TCM), a balanced diet is considered essential to maintain good health and prevent illnesses. TCM nutrition focuses on promoting health and preventing diseases by consuming foods that support the body's natural functions. Here are some foods that have been identified in TCM as particularly beneficial for cognitive function.

Leafy greens

Leafy greens such as spinach, kale, and collard greens are packed with vitamins and minerals such as iron, folate, and vitamins A and C. These nutrients play an important role in brain health, including cognitive function. Iron, for example, is essential for transporting oxygen to the brain, while folate and vitamin B12 are necessary for healthy nerve function.

Nuts and seeds

Nuts and seeds such as walnuts, almonds, and pumpkin seeds are excellent sources of omega-3 fatty acids, which are crucial for brain health. Omega-3 fatty acids are essential for building cell membranes in the brain, and studies have shown that they may help improve memory and cognitive function.

Berries

Berries such as blueberries, blackberries, and raspberries are high in antioxidants, which help protect the brain from oxidative stress. Studies have shown that eating berries regularly can improve cognitive function, including memory.

Whole grains

Whole grains such as brown rice, quinoa, and oatmeal are rich in complex carbohydrates, which provide the brain with a steady supply of energy. Additionally, whole grains are a good source of B vitamins, which are essential for healthy nerve function.

Fish

Fish such as salmon, tuna, and sardines are rich in omega-3 fatty acids, which as mentioned earlier, are important for brain health. Studies have also shown that eating fish regularly can help prevent cognitive decline in older adults.

Turmeric

Turmeric is a spice that has been used in TCM for centuries. It contains a compound called curcumin, which has been shown to have anti-inflammatory properties. Inflammation in the brain has been linked to cognitive decline, so consuming turmeric may help improve cognitive function.

Green tea

Green tea contains a compound called catechin, which has been shown to have neuroprotective effects. Studies have shown that drinking green tea regularly can help improve cognitive function and reduce the risk of developing cognitive impairments.

Eggs

Eggs are an excellent source of choline, a nutrient that is essential for healthy brain function. Choline is involved in the production of acetylcholine, a neurotransmitter that is important for memory and cognitive function.

Chapter Thirty

Food Allergies and Sensitivities in TCM Nutrition

Food allergies and sensitivities have become a widespread concern in recent years. Traditional Chinese Medicine (TCM) recognizes the importance of food in maintaining health and wellbeing, and it also acknowledges the impact that certain foods can have on the body. In TCM, food allergies and sensitivities are seen as imbalances in the body, and they are treated through a combination of dietary adjustments and herbal remedies.

TCM views food allergies and sensitivities as a result of imbalances in the body's energy, or Qi. These imbalances can be caused by a variety of factors, including genetics, emotional stress, and dietary habits. When the body's Qi is disrupted, it can lead to digestive issues, skin problems, fatigue, and other symptoms.

One of the primary ways that TCM addresses food allergies and sensitivities is through the concept of the "Five Elements." In TCM, each element corresponds to specific organs and bodily functions, and imbalances in these elements can lead to various health issues, including food allergies and sensitivities.

The Five Elements are Wood, Fire, Earth, Metal, and Water. Each element is associated with specific foods, flavors, and cooking techniques. By understanding which elements are out of balance in the body, TCM practitioners can recommend dietary adjustments that help to restore balance and alleviate symptoms.

For example, if someone has a Wood element imbalance, they may be more prone to developing food allergies and sensitivities. Foods that are associated with the Wood element include sour and pungent flavors, as well as foods that are high in fat and protein. In this case, a TCM practitioner may recommend reducing or eliminating these types of foods from the diet and increasing foods that correspond to other elements, such as Earth or Metal.

Another way that TCM addresses food allergies and sensitivities is through the use of herbal remedies. TCM practitioners may recommend specific herbs or herbal formulas that can help to strengthen the digestive system, reduce inflammation, and support overall health.

TCM practitioners may also use acupuncture to help treat food allergies and sensitivities. Acupuncture involves the insertion of thin needles into specific points on the body to help regulate the flow of Qi. By stimulating specific points, acupuncture can help to reduce inflammation and alleviate symptoms associated with food allergies and sensitivities.

In addition to these TCM treatments, there are also practical steps that individuals can take to manage food allergies and sensitivities. For example, keeping a food diary can help to identify trigger foods and patterns of symptoms. Eliminating or reducing these trigger foods can help to alleviate symptoms and improve overall health.

It is also important to ensure that the diet is well-balanced and includes a variety of nutrient-dense foods. TCM emphasizes the importance of consuming foods that are in season and locally grown, as these foods are believed to be more energetically balanced and beneficial for overall health.

The TCM perspective on food allergies and sensitivities

Traditional Chinese Medicine (TCM) is an ancient system of healing that views the body as a whole, interconnected system. It recognizes that the foods we eat can impact our health in both positive and negative ways. While TCM does not have a specific concept of food allergies or sensitivities, it does recognize that some foods may not be suitable for certain individuals based on their constitution or health condition.

In TCM, the concept of constitution refers to a person's unique physical and mental characteristics, including their tendencies towards certain health conditions. It is believed that each individual has a specific constitution that influences their susceptibility to illness and their response to various treatments, including dietary recommendations. TCM also recognizes that different seasons and environments can impact our health and dietary needs.

According to TCM principles, a balanced diet should include a variety of foods that nourish the body and support its functions. This includes foods that are considered to have warming or cooling properties, which can help to balance the body's internal environment. Foods that are considered to have dampening or drying properties may also be recommended based on an individual's constitution and health condition.

TCM practitioners may also consider the concept of Qi, which refers to the body's vital energy, when making dietary recommendations. It is believed that certain foods can support the flow of Qi and promote overall health and wellbeing. Conversely, foods that are considered to be "Qi stagnant" or disruptive to the body's energy flow may be avoided.

In terms of food allergies and sensitivities, TCM may not have a specific concept of these conditions, but it does recognize that certain foods may not be suitable for certain individuals based on their constitution and health condition. For example, individuals with a tendency towards dampness may be advised to avoid foods that are considered to be dampening, such as dairy products and greasy or fried foods. Similarly, individuals with a tendency towards heat may be advised to avoid foods that are considered to be heating, such as spicy foods and alcohol.

TCM also recognizes the importance of food preparation and cooking methods. Certain cooking methods may be recommended based on an individual's constitution and health condition, as well as the properties of the foods being cooked. For example, slow-cooked soups and stews may be recommended for individuals with weak digestion or those who are recovering from illness, while lightly steamed vegetables may be recommended for individuals who are prone to dampness.

In TCM, the emphasis is on balance and harmony, both within the body and between the body and its environment. Dietary recommendations are tailored to the individual's unique constitution and health condition, as well as the season and environment. By following these principles, individuals can support their overall health and wellbeing, and potentially prevent or manage health conditions.

It is important to note that TCM should not be used as a replacement for medical treatment for food allergies or sensitivities. If an individual suspects they have a food allergy or sensitivity, they should consult with a healthcare professional for proper diagnosis and treatment.

Adapting TCM nutrition principles for those with food restrictions

Adapting Traditional Chinese Medicine (TCM) nutrition principles can be a challenge for individuals with food restrictions due to allergies or sensitivities. However, it is possible to incorporate TCM nutrition into a diet that accommodates these restrictions.

First, it is important to understand the TCM perspective on food allergies and sensitivities. TCM practitioners believe that food sensitivities and allergies result from imbalances in the body's energy or qi. For example, individuals with weak digestive systems may develop food sensitivities, as their bodies cannot properly digest certain foods. TCM also recognizes that the symptoms of food allergies and sensitivities vary greatly, from skin rashes to gastrointestinal distress.

In TCM, food is viewed not only as a source of nutrition but also as a form of medicine. Therefore, it is important to avoid foods that exacerbate the body's imbalances and instead consume foods that support the body's energy and promote healing.

Individuals with food restrictions due to allergies or sensitivities can still benefit from TCM nutrition principles by following some simple guidelines. Here are some tips to adapt TCM nutrition for those with food restrictions:

1. Consult with a TCM practitioner: Individuals with food allergies or sensitivities should consult with a TCM practitioner to identify their specific imbalances and receive personalized dietary recommendations. TCM practitioners can use diagnostic techniques, such as tongue and pulse diagnosis, to assess the body's energy and recommend specific foods and herbs to support healing.

2. Focus on whole foods: Individuals with food restrictions should focus on whole, unprocessed foods to ensure that they are getting the necessary nutrients for optimal health. Whole foods, such as fruits, vegetables, whole grains, and lean protein, are generally well-tolerated by most individuals and provide a wide range of vitamins and minerals.

3. Experiment with alternative protein sources: Many individuals with food allergies or sensitivities may need to avoid traditional protein sources, such as dairy and soy. However, there are many alternative protein sources that are compatible with TCM nutrition, such as quinoa, lentils, and hemp seeds.

4. Incorporate healing herbs: TCM emphasizes the use of herbs to support the body's energy and promote healing. Many herbs, such as ginger, turmeric, and licorice root, have anti-inflammatory and digestive properties that can support individuals with food allergies or sensitivities.

5. Avoid trigger foods: Individuals with food allergies or sensitivities should avoid trigger foods that exacerbate their symptoms. This may require some experimentation to identify which foods are problematic, but avoiding trigger foods can help to alleviate symptoms and promote healing.

Chapter Thirty-One

TCM Nutrition and Food Safety

Traditional Chinese Medicine (TCM) places great emphasis on the role of food in promoting health and preventing disease. However, as with any type of food, there are potential risks associated with consuming certain foods and it is important to consider food safety in TCM nutrition.

One of the key principles of TCM is that each person is unique and therefore, their nutritional needs will vary based on their individual constitution and health status. It is important to consider any allergies or sensitivities to foods, as well as any medications or supplements being taken, when creating a TCM nutrition plan.

Another important consideration is the quality and safety of the food being consumed. In TCM, food is viewed as a source of both nourishment and medicine. Therefore, it is important to choose foods that are grown and prepared in a safe and healthy manner. This includes avoiding foods that are contaminated with pesticides, heavy metals, and other toxins.

To ensure food safety, it is important to choose foods that are fresh and properly stored. Foods that are past their expiration date or have been stored at improper temperatures should be avoided. It is also important to properly clean and prepare foods to prevent the spread of bacteria and other harmful microorganisms.

In addition to food safety considerations, there are also certain foods and preparations that should be avoided or limited in TCM nutrition. For example, TCM places great emphasis on balance and moderation in all aspects of life, including diet. Therefore, it is important to avoid over-consumption of certain foods, such as greasy or fatty foods, which can contribute to dampness and phlegm in the body.

Another consideration in TCM nutrition is the use of food as medicine. While certain foods can be used to support the body's natural healing processes, it is important to use caution when using food as medicine. Some foods, such as herbs and spices, can be potent and should only be used under the guidance of a qualified TCM practitioner.

When choosing foods for a TCM nutrition plan, it is important to focus on whole, nutrient-dense foods that are rich in vitamins, minerals, and other beneficial compounds. This includes a variety of fruits, vegetables, whole grains, lean proteins, and healthy fats. By focusing on these nutrient-dense foods, individuals can support their overall health and well-being while reducing their risk of disease.

In addition to choosing nutrient-dense foods, it is also important to pay attention to how foods are prepared. In TCM, cooking methods are viewed as an important aspect of food therapy. For example, boiling or steaming vegetables can help to retain their nutrients and make them easier to digest, while deep-frying or sautéing can add excess fat and create an overly greasy dish.

The importance of food safety in TCM

Traditional Chinese Medicine (TCM) emphasizes the importance of maintaining a healthy diet for overall wellbeing, including the prevention and treatment of disease. However, the quality and safety of the foods we consume can have a significant impact on our health. In TCM, food safety is a crucial factor to consider in creating a healthy and balanced diet.

The concept of food safety in TCM includes not only avoiding contamination by pathogens but also avoiding foods that are potentially harmful to the body. For example, TCM recognizes that certain foods may be energetically "hot" or "cold," and consuming too much of either can lead to imbalances in the body's systems.

Additionally, TCM recognizes that individuals may have different constitutional types and unique health concerns that require specific dietary recommendations. For example, someone with a weak digestive system may need to avoid certain foods that are difficult to digest, while someone with a deficiency in Qi (life force energy) may need to consume foods that help boost Qi levels.

In TCM, the quality of the food we eat is also important. The ideal food is one that is fresh, in season, and locally sourced. Foods that have been heavily processed, preserved with chemicals, or contain artificial additives may not be as beneficial for our health. TCM also emphasizes the importance of preparing food in a way that preserves its nutritional value, such as steaming or lightly cooking vegetables instead of boiling or frying them.

In recent years, food safety concerns have become increasingly important in TCM. Contamination of food by chemicals, heavy metals, and other environmental toxins can have detrimental effects on health, and TCM practitioners emphasize the importance of sourcing high-quality, safe food. Additionally, there have been reports of food fraud, where lower quality or even counterfeit ingredients are used in food products, which can compromise their safety and effectiveness.

One example of food safety concerns in TCM is the use of Chinese herbal medicines. While these remedies can be powerful tools for healing, there have been reports of contamination with heavy metals, pesticides, and other toxins. TCM practitioners must be careful to source high-quality herbs from reputable suppliers and ensure that they are properly tested and processed.

To ensure food safety in TCM, it is important to follow certain guidelines. First, choose fresh, whole foods that are locally sourced and in season. Whenever possible, choose organic or sustainably produced foods to minimize exposure to harmful chemicals and pesticides. Avoid heavily processed foods and those with artificial additives.

It is also important to properly store and prepare food to minimize the risk of contamination. Wash fruits and vegetables thoroughly before eating, and store food in airtight containers to prevent the growth of harmful bacteria. Use proper food handling techniques, such as separating raw meat from other foods and cooking meat to the appropriate temperature.

Safe food handling and storage practices

Safe food handling and storage practices are critical to ensuring that our food is safe to eat and free from harmful contaminants. In Traditional Chinese Medicine (TCM), food is not only seen as a source of nourishment, but also as a form of medicine. This means that it is essential to handle and store food properly to preserve its healing properties and prevent foodborne illnesses.

The first step to safe food handling is to ensure that all surfaces, utensils, and hands are clean before preparing food. This can be achieved by washing hands with soap and warm water for at least 20 seconds, washing utensils and cutting boards with hot, soapy water after each use, and wiping down surfaces with a sanitizing solution.

In TCM, it is believed that different types of food have different energetic properties, and therefore should be stored separately. For example, pungent and spicy foods should be stored separately from sweet foods, as they can easily absorb each other's flavors and energies. Additionally, food should be stored in a cool, dry place to prevent spoilage and contamination.

Another important aspect of safe food handling is proper cooking and reheating. Meat, poultry, and fish should be cooked to their recommended internal temperatures to kill any harmful bacteria. Leftovers should be reheated to a temperature of 165°F (74°C) to ensure that any bacteria are destroyed.

In TCM, it is believed that the way in which food is prepared and cooked can also affect its energetic properties. For example, boiling is believed to reduce the energetic properties of food, while steaming and stir-frying are believed to preserve them. This means that it is important to choose cooking methods that are appropriate for the type of food being prepared to preserve its healing properties.

Proper food storage is also important for food safety. Foods should be stored in airtight containers to prevent contamination, and perishable foods should be refrigerated promptly. It is also important to monitor the temperature of the refrigerator and ensure that it is below 40°F (4°C) to prevent the growth of harmful bacteria.

In TCM, it is believed that the temperature of food can also affect its energetic properties. For example, foods that are cooked and served cold are believed to have a cooling effect on the body, while foods that are served warm are believed to have a warming effect. This means that it is important to consider the temperature of food when preparing and storing it to ensure that it is appropriate for the intended use.

Finally, it is important to be aware of food recalls and take appropriate action if necessary. If a food product has been recalled due to contamination, it should be discarded immediately. It is also important to stay informed about food safety issues and take steps to protect oneself and one's family.

In TCM, food is seen as an important aspect of health and healing. By following safe food handling and storage practices, we can ensure that the food we eat is safe and free from harmful contaminants. By taking care to preserve the energetic properties of food, we can also ensure that it provides the greatest possible benefit to our health and wellbeing.

Chapter Thirty-Two

Mindful Eating and TCM Nutrition

Mindful eating is a practice that emphasizes paying attention to our food and eating habits in a non-judgmental way. It involves being present in the moment, noticing the sensory experience of eating, and cultivating a deeper connection with the food we consume. Mindful eating has been gaining popularity in recent years as a tool for promoting better health and wellbeing, and it aligns with the principles of Traditional Chinese Medicine (TCM) nutrition.

TCM is a holistic system of healing that emphasizes the interconnectedness of mind, body, and spirit. According to TCM, the foods we eat can have a significant impact on our health, and the way we approach eating is just as important as the foods we choose to consume. Mindful eating is a key aspect of TCM nutrition, as it encourages individuals to approach food with intention, awareness, and appreciation.

In TCM, each food has its unique properties, flavors, and energies that can affect the body in different ways. By cultivating a deeper understanding of the foods we consume, we can make more informed choices about what we eat and how we prepare it. For example, TCM emphasizes the importance of consuming a variety of foods to support the body's overall health and balance.

One important aspect of TCM nutrition is the concept of Qi, or vital energy, that flows throughout the body. Different foods are believed to have different Qi properties, which can impact the flow of energy in the body. For example, warming foods like ginger and garlic are believed to help promote circulation and warmth, while cooling foods like cucumber and watermelon can help reduce excess heat in the body. By paying attention to the Qi properties of the foods we eat, we can better support the body's natural balance and harmony.

Another important aspect of TCM nutrition is the practice of eating according to the seasons. In TCM, the seasons are believed to have a significant impact on the body's energy and vitality, and different foods are recommended for different times of the year. For example, during the cold winter months, TCM recommends consuming warming foods like soups, stews, and roasted vegetables to help support the body's internal warmth. In the summer months, cooling foods like salads and fresh fruits are recommended to help regulate the body's temperature and energy.

Mindful eating is an important component of TCM nutrition because it encourages individuals to pay attention to their body's needs and respond appropriately. By being present and aware during mealtime, we can tune into our body's natural hunger and fullness cues, which can help prevent overeating and support healthy digestion. Mindful eating can also help us cultivate a deeper appreciation for the foods we consume and the role they play in supporting our overall health and wellbeing.

In addition to mindful eating, there are several other TCM nutrition practices that can help promote optimal health and wellbeing. These include:

1. Eating a variety of whole foods: TCM recommends consuming a wide range of whole, unprocessed foods to support the body's overall health and balance. This includes fruits, vegetables, whole grains, lean proteins, and healthy fats.

2. Cooking with intention: The way we prepare our food can impact its energy and nutritional properties. TCM recommends cooking with

intention and mindfulness to help preserve the foods' vital energy and nutrients.

3. Eating in moderation: TCM recommends consuming food in moderation to avoid overtaxing the digestive system and supporting healthy digestion.

4. Drinking warm water: TCM recommends drinking warm water throughout the day to help support digestion and circulation.

5. Avoiding processed foods: TCM recommends avoiding highly processed and refined foods, which can be difficult to digest and may lack vital nutrients and energy.

The role of mindfulness in TCM nutrition

Traditional Chinese Medicine (TCM) has long recognized the importance of mindfulness in maintaining overall health and wellness. Mindfulness is a state of awareness that involves paying attention to the present moment, without judgment or distraction. This practice has been shown to have a positive impact on mental and emotional well-being, as well as physical health. When it comes to TCM nutrition, mindfulness is an essential component for optimal health.

TCM emphasizes the importance of eating mindfully and being fully present while eating. Mindful eating is a practice that involves paying attention to the texture, flavor, aroma, and visual presentation of food. It also involves being aware of the body's hunger and fullness signals and eating only until satisfied, not until feeling stuffed.

In TCM, it is believed that digestion starts in the mouth. Chewing food thoroughly and savoring each bite can help stimulate the production of digestive enzymes and improve nutrient absorption. Eating too quickly or while distracted, such as while watching TV or scrolling through social media, can lead to overeating and poor digestion.

Another important aspect of mindful eating in TCM is the concept of food energetics. In TCM, foods are categorized based on their energetic properties, such as temperature, taste, and whether they have a warming or cooling effect on the body. Eating a balanced variety of foods with different energetic properties is believed to help maintain overall health and prevent disease.

For example, foods that are considered warming in TCM, such as ginger, garlic, and cinnamon, are thought to help improve circulation, boost metabolism, and reduce inflammation. Foods that are considered cooling, such as cucumber, watermelon, and mung bean, are thought to help clear heat and reduce inflammation.

In addition to being mindful while eating, TCM also emphasizes the importance of eating in a calm and peaceful environment. Eating in a rushed or stressful environment can lead to digestive problems and poor nutrient absorption. Eating in a relaxed and peaceful environment can help improve digestion and nutrient absorption, as well as promote a sense of calm and well-being.

TCM also encourages the consumption of whole, unprocessed foods, such as fruits, vegetables, whole grains, and lean proteins. These foods are nutrient-dense and are believed to support overall health and well-being. TCM also emphasizes the importance of eating a variety of colors, as different colors are associated with different nutrients and energetic properties.

Incorporating mindfulness into meal planning and preparation can also be beneficial for overall health and well-being. Taking the time to plan and prepare meals mindfully can help reduce stress and promote a sense of calm. Mindful meal planning can also help ensure a balanced and varied diet that supports overall health.

When it comes to TCM nutrition, mindfulness is an essential component for optimal health. Mindful eating and being fully present while eating can help improve digestion, nutrient absorption, and overall health. Eating in a calm and peaceful environment, choosing whole, unprocessed foods, and incorporating a variety of colors and energetic properties can also support optimal health and well-being.

Practicing mindful eating for better digestion and overall health

Practicing mindful eating is a powerful tool for improving digestion and overall health. Mindful eating is a practice rooted in traditional Chinese medicine (TCM) that emphasizes the importance of paying attention to the experience of eating, from the taste and texture of food to the sensation of fullness. By bringing awareness and intention to our meals, we can optimize digestion, reduce overeating, and improve our relationship with food.

In TCM, digestion is viewed as a critical foundation of health. Proper digestion is essential for nourishing the body and mind, while poor digestion can lead to a range of health issues. According to TCM, the digestive system plays a crucial role in transforming food into Qi, or life energy, which is then distributed throughout the body to support overall health and vitality.

To optimize digestion and support overall health, TCM emphasizes the importance of mindful eating. This involves taking time to appreciate the flavors and textures of food, chewing food thoroughly, and paying attention to feelings of fullness. By doing so, we can support the digestive system in breaking down and absorbing nutrients from our food more efficiently.

One simple practice for mindful eating is to eat without distractions. This means turning off the television, putting away the phone, and focusing entirely on the experience of eating. When we eat while distracted, we are more likely to overeat and less likely to be aware of our body's signals of fullness.

Another important aspect of mindful eating is chewing food thoroughly. Chewing breaks down food into smaller particles, making it easier for the digestive system to process. When we chew food thoroughly, we also release more nutrients from the food, which can enhance our overall nutritional intake.

In addition to eating mindfully, TCM also recommends eating in a relaxed and peaceful environment. This means avoiding stressful or emotionally charged situations while eating. When we eat in a calm and peaceful environment, we are more likely to be relaxed, which supports optimal digestion.

TCM also suggests eating regular meals at consistent times each day. This helps to regulate the digestive system and promote optimal digestion. Irregular eating habits can disrupt the digestive system, leading to issues like bloating, gas, and indigestion.

In terms of the types of foods to eat, TCM emphasizes a balanced diet that includes a variety of whole, nutrient-dense foods. This includes vegetables, fruits, whole grains, and lean protein sources. It is also important to avoid overly processed and refined foods, as these can be difficult for the digestive system to process.

TCM also recommends incorporating specific foods and herbs that are beneficial for digestion. For example, ginger is known for its anti-inflammatory properties and can help soothe the digestive system. Turmeric is another spice that can support digestive health, as it contains anti-inflammatory compounds and can stimulate bile production.

Incorporating probiotic-rich foods, like fermented vegetables and yogurt, can also support optimal digestion. Probiotics are beneficial bacteria that reside in the gut and support healthy digestion and immune function.

Chapter Thirty-Three

TCM Nutrition and Exercise

Traditional Chinese Medicine (TCM) emphasizes the importance of diet and exercise in maintaining good health. While diet and nutrition play a major role in TCM, exercise is also an essential component of a healthy lifestyle. TCM practitioners recommend incorporating exercise into one's daily routine to enhance overall health, prevent illness, and promote longevity.

1. TCM identifies two types of exercise: "hard" and "soft." Hard exercise refers to high-intensity activities such as weightlifting, running, or high-impact sports. Soft exercise, on the other hand, includes low-intensity activities such as walking, tai chi, and yoga. Both hard and soft exercises can be beneficial for the body, but the key is to find a balance that works for each individual.

In TCM, the body is viewed as a whole, with all parts interconnected and interdependent. Exercise is seen as a way to enhance the flow of qi, or vital energy, throughout the body. When the flow of qi is disrupted or blocked, it can lead to health problems. Exercise helps to move qi through the body and keep it flowing smoothly, promoting overall health and well-being.

In addition to promoting qi flow, exercise also strengthens the body, increases flexibility and mobility, and improves cardiovascular health. It can help to reduce stress and anxiety, improve sleep quality, and enhance mental clarity and focus.

When it comes to exercise and TCM nutrition, it's important to consider the individual's constitution and specific health needs. For example, a person with a weak constitution may benefit from gentle, low-impact exercises such as tai chi or yoga, while someone with a stronger constitution may benefit from more intense exercise such as running or weightlifting.

TCM nutrition also plays a role in supporting exercise and physical activity. Eating a healthy diet with balanced macronutrients (carbohydrates, protein, and fat) and a variety of micronutrients (vitamins and minerals) can provide the body with the energy and nutrients it needs to support physical activity.

Carbohydrates are the body's primary source of energy and are especially important for high-intensity exercise. Complex carbohydrates such as whole grains, fruits, and vegetables provide sustained energy throughout the day. Protein is important for muscle repair and recovery after exercise, and sources such as lean meats, legumes, and dairy products can help to support muscle growth and repair. Healthy fats such as those found in nuts, seeds, and avocados can provide energy and support heart health.

In addition to macronutrients, micronutrients such as iron, magnesium, and B vitamins are also important for exercise and physical activity. Iron is necessary for the production of hemoglobin, which carries oxygen in the blood, while magnesium is important for muscle and nerve function. B vitamins play a role in energy metabolism and can help to reduce fatigue and support mental clarity and focus.

The connection between diet and physical activity in TCM

Traditional Chinese Medicine (TCM) recognizes the importance of maintaining an active lifestyle for overall health and well-being. However, it is equally important to understand the connection between physical activity and diet in TCM. Diet is an integral part of TCM, and it is believed that the right foods can support the body during physical activity, enhance performance, and aid in recovery. Below we will explore the connection between diet and physical activity in TCM and how one can use TCM nutrition to enhance their exercise routine.

According to TCM, food is classified based on its energetic properties, such as temperature, flavor, and direction of movement. The energy of food is believed to interact with the body's energy, or Qi, to maintain balance and promote health. In TCM, a balanced diet is one that includes a variety of foods that are energetically balanced and supports the body's needs. For example, foods that are warming in nature are ideal for individuals who tend to feel cold, while cooling foods are recommended for those who tend to feel hot.

Physical activity is also an essential component of TCM. In TCM, physical activity is viewed as a means to promote the flow of Qi and blood throughout the body. When Qi and blood are flowing smoothly, the body can function optimally, and the risk of illness and disease is reduced. Additionally, physical activity is believed to strengthen the body's internal organs and improve overall vitality.

When it comes to exercise and physical activity, TCM recommends that individuals choose activities that are appropriate for their body type and constitution. For example, individuals with a weaker constitution may benefit from gentle exercises such as tai chi or yoga, while those with a stronger constitution may thrive with more intense exercise such as weightlifting or running.

Diet is an essential component of an individual's ability to engage in physical activity. In TCM, foods are classified based on their energetic properties, and it is recommended that individuals consume foods that are energetically balanced and support their body's needs. For example, individuals who engage in intense physical activity may benefit from consuming warming foods such as ginger, garlic, and cinnamon, which are believed to promote circulation and increase energy. Additionally, it is recommended to consume foods that are high in protein and healthy fats to support muscle repair and recovery.

Another important consideration for TCM nutrition and physical activity is timing. In TCM, it is believed that consuming foods at the right time can enhance the body's ability to utilize the energy provided by food. For example, consuming a meal high in carbohydrates before engaging in physical activity can provide the body with the energy it needs to perform at its best. Additionally, consuming foods that are high in protein and healthy fats after physical activity can aid in muscle repair and recovery.

In TCM, it is also important to consider the preparation and cooking methods of food. It is believed that certain cooking methods can enhance the energetic properties of food and make it easier for the body to digest. For example, slow cooking methods such as stewing and simmering can help break down tough fibers in meat and make it easier for the body to absorb nutrients.

Furthermore, TCM emphasizes the importance of listening to the body's needs during physical activity. It is recommended that individuals pay attention to how their body responds to different types of physical activity and adjust their diet accordingly. For example, if an individual experiences muscle soreness after engaging in weightlifting, consuming foods that are high in anti-inflammatory properties such as turmeric, ginger, and omega-3 fatty acids can aid in recovery.

Foods that support exercise and recovery

Foods play a crucial role in providing the body with the necessary nutrients for optimal physical activity and exercise performance. In Traditional Chinese Medicine (TCM), food is seen as a powerful tool for supporting the body's natural processes and promoting overall health and wellness. By incorporating TCM nutrition principles, individuals can choose foods that support their exercise goals and promote a healthy recovery process.

The TCM perspective on exercise emphasizes the importance of balancing yin and yang energies in the body. Yin and yang are opposing forces that exist in everything, including the human body. Yin represents the cooler, more passive aspects of the body, while yang represents the warmer, more active aspects. In TCM, optimal health is achieved by maintaining a balance between these two energies.

When it comes to exercise, TCM recommends balancing yang energy with yin-nourishing foods to prevent depletion and promote a healthy recovery process. Yang-nourishing foods, on the other hand, can be beneficial for increasing energy levels and promoting optimal performance.

One key TCM nutrition principle for supporting exercise and physical activity is to consume foods that are easily digestible. When the body is engaged in physical activity, it diverts blood flow away from the digestive system to the muscles. Consuming heavy, difficult-to-digest foods before exercise can lead to discomfort, bloating, and decreased performance. Instead, individuals should choose light, nutrient-dense foods that can be easily absorbed and utilized by the body.

Another important TCM nutrition principle for exercise is to choose foods that are rich in qi, the vital energy that circulates throughout the body. Qi is believed to be responsible for maintaining overall health and vitality, as well as supporting the body's natural healing processes. Foods that are rich in qi include whole grains, vegetables, and fruits.

Protein is also crucial for supporting physical activity and exercise. In TCM, protein is believed to nourish the muscles and support the body's natural repair processes. Good sources of protein include lean meats, fish, legumes, and nuts.

In addition to macronutrients, micronutrients are also important for supporting physical activity and exercise. Certain vitamins and minerals, such as vitamin C, vitamin E, and magnesium, have been shown to support muscle recovery and prevent oxidative stress in the body. Foods that are rich in these nutrients include leafy greens, nuts, seeds, and berries.

Hydration is also key for optimal exercise performance and recovery. In TCM, it is recommended to consume warm or room temperature fluids, as cold fluids can disrupt the body's natural balance of yin and yang energies. Water, herbal teas, and bone broths are all good options for staying hydrated during and after exercise.

When it comes to recovery, TCM nutrition principles emphasize the importance of consuming foods that nourish yin energy and support the body's natural healing processes. Yin-nourishing foods, such as leafy greens, fruits, and root vegetables, can help to restore balance in the body and promote recovery.

Chapter Thirty-Four

The Role of TCM Nutrition in Integrative Healthcare

Traditional Chinese Medicine (TCM) is an ancient medical system that has been used for thousands of years to promote health and treat illness. TCM includes a wide range of practices, including acupuncture, herbal medicine, massage, and dietary therapy. TCM dietary therapy, also known as TCM nutrition, is an important component of TCM practice that focuses on using food as medicine to maintain health and prevent disease.

Integrative healthcare, which combines conventional medicine with complementary and alternative therapies, is becoming increasingly popular. TCM nutrition is a valuable addition to integrative healthcare because it can help address many health concerns that conventional medicine may not fully address. Below we will discuss the role of TCM nutrition in integrative healthcare, including its benefits and potential drawbacks.

TCM nutrition emphasizes the importance of eating a balanced diet based on an individual's constitution, environment, and specific health concerns. This approach recognizes that food has energetic properties that can either support or hinder the body's natural functions. TCM nutrition also emphasizes the importance of cooking methods and food preparation, such as slow cooking, steaming, and fermentation, to enhance the nutritional value of food and make it easier for the body to digest.

One of the benefits of TCM nutrition in integrative healthcare is its ability to address chronic health conditions that may not respond well to conventional medical treatments. For example, TCM nutrition can help regulate blood sugar levels in individuals with type 2 diabetes by recommending foods that support insulin sensitivity, such as bitter melon, cinnamon, and green tea. TCM nutrition can also help manage autoimmune conditions, such as rheumatoid arthritis and lupus, by recommending anti-inflammatory foods, such as ginger, turmeric, and leafy greens.

TCM nutrition can also be used to support cancer treatment and recovery. TCM practitioners use food therapy to help alleviate chemotherapy side effects, boost the immune system, and promote overall wellness. For example, TCM nutrition may recommend foods such as mushrooms, seaweed, and fermented foods to support immune function during cancer treatment.

Another benefit of TCM nutrition in integrative healthcare is its focus on prevention. TCM nutrition emphasizes the importance of a balanced diet and lifestyle to maintain health and prevent disease. By identifying and addressing imbalances in the body early on, TCM nutrition can prevent the development of chronic health conditions such as cardiovascular disease, type 2 diabetes, and autoimmune disorders.

However, TCM nutrition is not without its potential drawbacks. One of the challenges of TCM nutrition is the lack of scientific research to support its claims. While there is some evidence to suggest that certain foods and dietary practices used in TCM nutrition can be beneficial for health, more rigorous scientific studies are needed to confirm these claims.

Another challenge of TCM nutrition is the potential for adverse reactions and interactions with conventional medications. Some herbs and foods used in TCM nutrition may interact with prescription medications, and individuals with certain health conditions may need to avoid or modify their diets to prevent adverse reactions.

The benefits of combining TCM nutrition with Western medicine

Traditional Chinese Medicine (TCM) has been used for centuries to maintain health and treat various health conditions. One aspect of TCM that has gained popularity in recent years is TCM nutrition, which involves using food and herbs to support health and prevent and treat illness. While TCM nutrition has been traditionally used on its own, it can also be integrated with Western medicine to provide a more comprehensive approach to healthcare. Below we will explore the benefits of combining TCM nutrition with Western medicine.

One of the main benefits of integrating TCM nutrition with Western medicine is that it can lead to a more personalized and holistic approach to healthcare. Western medicine tends to focus on treating symptoms and diseases, often through medications or surgery. While these treatments can be effective, they may not address the root cause of the problem or take into account the individual's unique constitution and lifestyle factors. TCM, on the other hand, takes a holistic approach that considers the whole person, including their physical, emotional, and spiritual health. By combining TCM nutrition with Western medicine, healthcare providers can create a more personalized treatment plan that takes into account the individual's unique needs and preferences.

Another benefit of integrating TCM nutrition with Western medicine is that it can enhance the effectiveness of treatments. TCM nutrition can be used to support the body's natural healing processes and enhance the effects of medications and other treatments. For example, certain foods and herbs can be used to reduce inflammation and support the immune system, which can be beneficial for individuals with chronic conditions such as autoimmune diseases. TCM nutrition can also be used to help manage side effects of medications, such as digestive issues or fatigue.

In addition to enhancing the effectiveness of treatments, integrating TCM nutrition with Western medicine can also help prevent disease and promote long-term health. TCM nutrition emphasizes the importance of eating a balanced diet that includes a variety of whole foods and herbs. This can help prevent nutrient deficiencies and support overall health and vitality. Additionally, TCM nutrition can be used to address imbalances in the body that may lead to chronic health conditions. For example, certain foods and herbs can be used to support digestive health, which can prevent the development of digestive disorders such as irritable bowel syndrome or inflammatory bowel disease.

Integrating TCM nutrition with Western medicine can also provide a more patient-centered approach to healthcare. TCM nutrition emphasizes the importance of listening to the body and paying attention to its needs. By incorporating TCM nutrition into their practice, healthcare providers can encourage patients to take an active role in their own healthcare and empower them to make choices that support their health and well-being. This can lead to better patient satisfaction and a greater sense of control over one's health.

Finally, integrating TCM nutrition with Western medicine can also provide a more cost-effective approach to healthcare. TCM nutrition emphasizes the use of whole foods and herbs, which are often less expensive than medications and other treatments. Additionally, TCM nutrition can be used to prevent the development of chronic health conditions, which can save individuals and healthcare systems money in the long run.

Working with healthcare professionals to optimize your TCM nutrition plan

Traditional Chinese Medicine (TCM) nutrition is a holistic approach to health and wellness that focuses on using food as medicine to promote healing and prevent illness. It is based on the concept of Qi, or vital energy, which flows throughout the body and is influenced by various factors, including diet and lifestyle.

When it comes to developing a TCM nutrition plan, working with a healthcare professional can be an important part of the process. A qualified TCM practitioner or integrative healthcare provider can help you identify imbalances in your body and design a personalized nutrition plan to address your unique needs.

One of the benefits of working with a healthcare professional is that they can help you navigate the complexities of TCM nutrition. TCM theory can be complex, and it may be difficult to know which foods are appropriate for your specific health concerns. For example, certain foods may be beneficial for someone with a Yin deficiency, while other foods may be more appropriate for someone with a Yang deficiency. A healthcare professional can help you understand which foods are appropriate for your individual needs and create a balanced diet that promotes optimal health and wellness.

Another benefit of working with a healthcare professional is that they can help you avoid potential interactions between TCM herbs and Western medications. Many TCM herbs have been used for centuries to treat a variety of health conditions, but they can also interact with certain medications, such as blood thinners or antidepressants. A qualified healthcare professional can help you identify potential interactions and develop a safe and effective TCM nutrition plan.

In addition, working with a healthcare professional can help you track your progress and make adjustments to your nutrition plan as needed. TCM nutrition is not a one-size-fits-all approach, and what works for one person may not work for another. By working with a healthcare professional, you can monitor your progress and make changes to your nutrition plan based on your individual response.

When seeking a healthcare professional to help with your TCM nutrition plan, it is important to find someone who is qualified and experienced in both TCM and Western medicine. Look for a licensed acupuncturist or integrative healthcare provider who has experience working with TCM nutrition and can provide a comprehensive assessment of your health needs.

In addition, it is important to communicate openly and honestly with your healthcare professional about your health concerns, lifestyle, and dietary habits. This will help them design a personalized TCM nutrition plan that is tailored to your unique needs and goals.

Finally, it is important to remember that TCM nutrition is just one part of a holistic approach to health and wellness. In addition to eating a balanced diet, it is important to get regular exercise, practice stress-reducing techniques, and get enough restorative sleep. By incorporating these practices into your daily life and working with a qualified healthcare professional, you can optimize your TCM nutrition plan and promote optimal health and wellness for the long-term.

Chapter Thirty-Five

TCM Nutrition for a Sustainable and Ethical Lifestyle

Traditional Chinese Medicine (TCM) is a holistic system of healthcare that has been practiced for thousands of years. In TCM, food is considered a form of medicine that can be used to prevent and treat various health conditions. TCM nutrition emphasizes the importance of consuming whole, unprocessed foods that are rich in nutrients and free of harmful chemicals. In addition, TCM nutrition also takes into account the ethical and environmental impact of food choices. Below we will discuss how TCM nutrition can help promote a sustainable and ethical lifestyle.

Sustainability is a growing concern in modern society, and it is important to consider the environmental impact of our food choices. TCM nutrition promotes the consumption of whole, unprocessed foods that are locally sourced and in season. This not only helps reduce the carbon footprint of our food choices but also ensures that we consume fresh and nutrient-rich foods that are in harmony with nature. In TCM, it is believed that consuming foods that are in season can help balance the body's energy and promote optimal health. For example, during the summer months, we should consume more cooling foods such as watermelon and cucumber to help balance the body's energy and prevent heat-related illnesses.

In addition to promoting sustainable food choices, TCM nutrition also emphasizes the importance of ethical considerations when it comes to food consumption. TCM recognizes the interconnectedness of all living beings and promotes the concept of "food as medicine." This means that we should respect the source of our food and consume it with gratitude and mindfulness. TCM encourages the consumption of foods that are raised and harvested in ethical and sustainable ways. For example, choosing grass-fed, pasture-raised meat or wild-caught fish can help reduce the negative impact of animal agriculture on the environment and support the humane treatment of animals.

TCM also recognizes the importance of food quality and purity. In TCM, it is believed that consuming foods that are free of harmful chemicals and additives is essential for promoting optimal health. This means choosing foods that are organic and free of pesticides, hormones, and other harmful substances. TCM also promotes the consumption of foods that are minimally processed and free of artificial flavors, colors, and preservatives.

Incorporating TCM nutrition principles into our daily lives can be a powerful tool for promoting a sustainable and ethical lifestyle. Some tips for integrating TCM nutrition into our daily routines include:

Choosing whole, unprocessed foods that are locally sourced and in season.

Consuming foods that are raised and harvested in ethical and sustainable ways, such as choosing grass-fed, pasture-raised meat or wild-caught fish.

Choosing foods that are free of harmful chemicals and additives, such as organic produce and minimally processed foods.

Consuming foods mindfully and with gratitude, recognizing the interconnectedness of all living beings and the importance of food as medicine.

Supporting local farmers and producers who prioritize sustainability and ethical practices.

The importance of sustainability and ethics in TCM nutrition

Traditional Chinese Medicine (TCM) is a holistic system of medicine that recognizes the interconnection between the human body and nature. TCM places great importance on the concept of Qi, the vital energy that flows through the body, and how it is influenced by our environment, including the food we eat. As such, TCM nutrition is not only concerned with the nutritional value of food but also its impact on the environment and society. In recent years, there has been an increasing awareness of the importance of sustainable and ethical food choices, and TCM nutrition can play a valuable role in guiding us towards a more conscious way of eating.

The principles of TCM nutrition are based on the concept of Yin and Yang, two opposing but complementary forces that exist in the body and in nature. Yin represents coolness, moisture, and stillness, while Yang represents warmth, dryness, and movement. In TCM, the goal is to maintain a balance between these two opposing forces, and food is categorized as either Yin or Yang, depending on its properties. For example, Yin foods include fruits, vegetables, and fish, while Yang foods include meats, nuts, and grains.

Sustainable and ethical food choices align with TCM principles because they prioritize the balance between the body and the environment. Sustainable food choices consider the environmental impact of food production, including the use of resources such as water, land, and energy. Ethical food choices consider the social impact of food production, including the treatment of animals and workers.

One of the ways to achieve a sustainable and ethical TCM nutrition plan is to choose locally sourced and seasonal foods. Eating locally reduces the carbon footprint of transportation, and seasonal foods are more likely to be grown in a sustainable manner. Eating a variety of fruits and vegetables from local farmers' markets can also provide a range of Yin and Yang foods to maintain balance in the body.

Another important consideration is the quality of the food we eat. TCM emphasizes the importance of whole, unprocessed foods that are free from harmful additives and chemicals. Choosing organic produce and meats from ethical sources can also ensure that the food we eat is free from harmful pesticides and hormones. In TCM, food is also prepared and cooked in a way that maximizes its nutritional value, such as steaming, boiling, or stir-frying.

TCM nutrition also emphasizes the importance of mindful eating, which involves being present and fully engaged with the eating experience. This includes paying attention to the taste, texture, and aroma of the food, as well as listening to the body's hunger and satiety cues. Mindful eating can help us make more conscious food choices and prevent overeating, which can contribute to both personal and environmental health.

Finally, TCM nutrition also emphasizes the use of medicinal foods and herbs, which have been used for centuries to support health and healing. These foods and herbs are believed to have specific properties that can nourish and balance the body, support the immune system, and promote longevity. Some examples of medicinal foods and herbs include ginger, turmeric, goji berries, and shiitake mushrooms.

Choosing eco-friendly and ethically sourced foods

Choosing eco-friendly and ethically sourced foods is not only important for the health of our planet, but it is also a crucial aspect of TCM nutrition. Traditional Chinese Medicine emphasizes the interconnectivity of all things and recognizes the role of environmental factors in our health and well-being. Therefore, making conscious choices about the food we eat can have a significant impact on both our own health and the health of the planet.

One of the key principles of TCM nutrition is that we should eat foods that are in harmony with our environment and the seasons. This means choosing foods that are grown locally and in season. Not only does this reduce the environmental impact of transporting food long distances, but it also ensures that we are eating foods that are at the peak of their nutritional value. Eating seasonally also supports local farmers and helps to strengthen local food systems.

Another important aspect of eco-friendly and ethical food choices is to consider the methods of production. For example, choosing organic foods can help to reduce exposure to harmful pesticides and herbicides, which can have negative impacts on both human and environmental health. It is also important to consider the treatment of animals in the food production process. Choosing animal products that are sourced from free-range or pasture-raised animals can help to reduce the environmental impact of factory farming and improve animal welfare.

In addition to considering the source of our food, it is important to think about the packaging and waste associated with our food choices. Single-use plastics are a major contributor to environmental pollution and can harm wildlife and ecosystems. Choosing foods that are minimally packaged or packaged in biodegradable or compostable materials can help to reduce our environmental impact. Additionally, reducing food waste by planning meals, composting food scraps, and choosing foods with longer shelf lives can help to reduce our carbon footprint and support a more sustainable food system.

When it comes to TCM nutrition, the principles of eco-friendliness and ethical sourcing are closely tied to the concept of Qi, or vital energy. Foods that are grown and produced in harmony with nature are believed to contain a higher level of Qi and are therefore more beneficial to our health. By making conscious choices about the foods we eat, we can not only support our own health and well-being but also contribute to a more sustainable and ethical food system.

Chapter Thirty-Six

The Future of TCM Nutrition

Traditional Chinese Medicine (TCM) has been a crucial part of healthcare in China for thousands of years. With its focus on balance and harmony within the body, TCM has evolved into a complete system of medicine that includes various modalities such as acupuncture, herbal medicine, and nutrition. TCM nutrition, in particular, has become increasingly popular in recent years, with more and more people turning to it for its holistic approach to health and wellness. As we look to the future, there are exciting developments in the field of TCM nutrition that are set to transform the way we approach health and wellness.

One of the most promising trends in TCM nutrition is the integration of technology into the practice. Technology is being used to create personalized nutrition plans that take into account an individual's unique needs and health goals. This is done through the use of AI-powered algorithms that analyze an individual's health data and make recommendations based on their specific needs. For example, if someone has high blood pressure, the algorithm may recommend foods that are rich in potassium and low in sodium, such as leafy greens and bananas. By using technology to create personalized nutrition plans, TCM practitioners can provide more effective and targeted treatment to their patients.

Another trend in TCM nutrition is the emphasis on whole foods and plant-based diets. TCM nutrition has always placed a strong emphasis on the importance of food as medicine. However, with the rise of processed and packaged foods, it has become increasingly difficult to maintain a whole foods-based diet. To address this issue, TCM practitioners are encouraging their patients to adopt a plant-based diet that is rich in whole foods. This approach not only helps to prevent chronic diseases such as heart disease and diabetes but also supports the body's natural healing process.

The use of functional foods is another exciting trend in TCM nutrition. Functional foods are those that have specific health benefits beyond basic nutrition. For example, foods that are high in antioxidants, such as blueberries, can help to reduce inflammation and prevent oxidative damage to the body. In TCM, functional foods have been used for centuries to treat a range of conditions, from digestive disorders to respiratory issues. As we continue to learn more about the health benefits of different foods, we can expect to see more functional foods being incorporated into TCM nutrition plans.

One area where TCM nutrition is already making a big impact is in the treatment of chronic diseases. Chronic diseases such as diabetes, heart disease, and cancer are a major health concern worldwide, and they are often treated with medications that can have serious side effects. TCM nutrition offers a natural and holistic approach to the treatment of these diseases, with a focus on lifestyle changes such as diet and exercise. By working with a TCM practitioner, patients with chronic diseases can learn how to manage their symptoms and improve their overall health and quality of life.

Finally, TCM nutrition is also becoming more accessible to people around the world. As interest in TCM grows, more and more people are seeking out TCM practitioners for guidance on nutrition and other aspects of health and wellness. This has led to the development of online courses and educational programs that make it easier for people to learn about

TCM nutrition and incorporate it into their lives. As TCM becomes more mainstream, we can expect to see even greater access to TCM nutrition resources and support.

The evolution of TCM nutrition in modern society

Traditional Chinese Medicine (TCM) is an ancient system of healthcare that has been in practice for thousands of years. TCM encompasses various practices, including acupuncture, herbal medicine, and TCM nutrition. TCM nutrition is based on the principles of balancing the body's energy, or Qi, through the food we eat. Over the years, TCM nutrition has evolved and adapted to modern society's needs and demands.

One of the main reasons for the evolution of TCM nutrition is the changing dietary habits of modern society. With the availability of processed foods, fast food, and the ease of access to food, people's diets have changed significantly. This has led to an increase in health problems such as obesity, diabetes, and heart disease. TCM nutrition has adapted to these changes by focusing on promoting healthier food choices and educating people about the importance of a balanced diet.

Another factor that has influenced the evolution of TCM nutrition is the growing interest in holistic and alternative healthcare practices. People are becoming more aware of the link between their diet and their overall health and are seeking natural ways to improve their well-being. TCM nutrition is gaining popularity as an effective way to improve health and prevent illness.

The advancement in scientific research has also contributed to the evolution of TCM nutrition. Modern science has helped to validate the effectiveness of TCM nutrition and its principles. Studies have shown that some TCM foods and herbs have medicinal properties that can help prevent and treat certain health conditions. This has led to the integration of TCM nutrition into mainstream healthcare practices.

Moreover, the rise of sustainable and ethical food practices has also impacted the evolution of TCM nutrition. As people become more conscious of the impact of their food choices on the environment and animal welfare, there is a growing demand for eco-friendly and ethically sourced foods. TCM nutrition emphasizes the importance of natural, whole foods that are free from chemicals and pesticides, making it a perfect fit for those seeking a more sustainable and ethical lifestyle.

The future of TCM nutrition is promising, with the continued integration of TCM into mainstream healthcare practices. The integration of TCM nutrition into conventional healthcare practices can help provide more comprehensive care for patients, promoting better health outcomes. As more research is conducted on TCM nutrition, we can expect to learn more about the health benefits of TCM foods and herbs, leading to even more integration of TCM into modern healthcare practices.

In addition, the use of technology is also expected to play a significant role in the evolution of TCM nutrition. The development of mobile apps and wearable devices that track food intake and nutritional status can help people make better food choices and promote healthier eating habits. These technological advancements can also help people to monitor their progress and track the effectiveness of their TCM nutrition plan.

Emerging research and trends in TCM nutrition

Traditional Chinese Medicine (TCM) has a rich history of using nutrition as a key aspect of healing and disease prevention. Today, TCM nutrition continues to gain attention and interest from researchers, practitioners, and the public. With a growing interest in integrative medicine and alternative therapies, TCM nutrition is becoming more widely accepted as a viable approach to achieving optimal health.

Emerging research in TCM nutrition is focused on exploring the therapeutic benefits of specific foods, herbs, and dietary patterns for a range of health conditions. One area of research is the role of TCM nutrition in managing chronic diseases such as diabetes, cardiovascular disease, and cancer. Studies have found that TCM dietary interventions may improve blood sugar control, reduce inflammation, and improve quality of life in cancer patients.

Another area of interest is the impact of TCM nutrition on mental health. Research has shown that certain foods and herbs traditionally used in TCM may have a positive effect on anxiety, depression, and stress. For example, studies have found that the amino acid theanine, found in green tea, may promote relaxation and reduce stress.

There is also growing interest in the use of TCM nutrition for weight management. TCM practitioners have long recognized the connection between nutrition and weight management and have developed dietary guidelines and herbal formulas for promoting weight loss. Research has shown that TCM dietary interventions may be effective for reducing body weight, body mass index (BMI), and waist circumference.

One emerging trend in TCM nutrition is the use of personalized nutrition. TCM recognizes that each person is unique and requires an individualized approach to nutrition. This approach takes into account a person's constitution, current health status, and specific health concerns. Personalized nutrition involves the use of dietary assessments, lab tests, and other diagnostic tools to develop a tailored nutrition plan for each individual.

Another trend is the integration of TCM nutrition with modern nutritional science. Researchers are beginning to explore the mechanisms of action of TCM foods and herbs and to identify their active compounds. This research is shedding light on the potential therapeutic benefits of TCM nutrition and helping to bridge the gap between traditional and modern approaches to nutrition.

In addition to research, there are also emerging trends in the practice of TCM nutrition. One trend is the use of food therapy as a primary mode of treatment. Food therapy involves the use of whole foods and culinary herbs to treat and prevent disease. TCM practitioners may develop personalized food therapy plans for their patients, which include specific foods and cooking techniques tailored to the individual's needs.

Another trend is the use of TCM nutrition in conjunction with other TCM therapies such as acupuncture and herbal medicine. TCM recognizes the importance of a holistic approach to health, and combining nutrition with other therapies may enhance their effectiveness.

* 9 7 8 1 7 7 6 9 6 8 1 4 5 *

SD - #0031 - 140926 - C0 - 229/152/14 - PB - 9781776968145 - Matt Lamination